Michael L. Jo

Divine Creations

The Daniel Fast Experience

Fasting to Renew Your Spirit and Strengthen Your Body

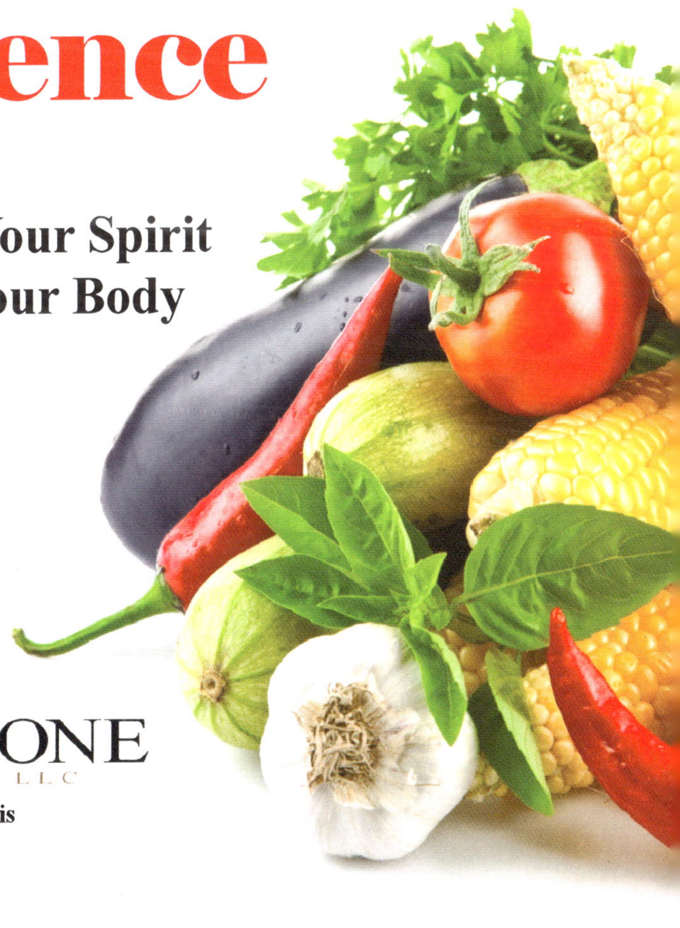

BROWNSTONE
PUBLICATIONS, LLC
Bloomington, Illinois

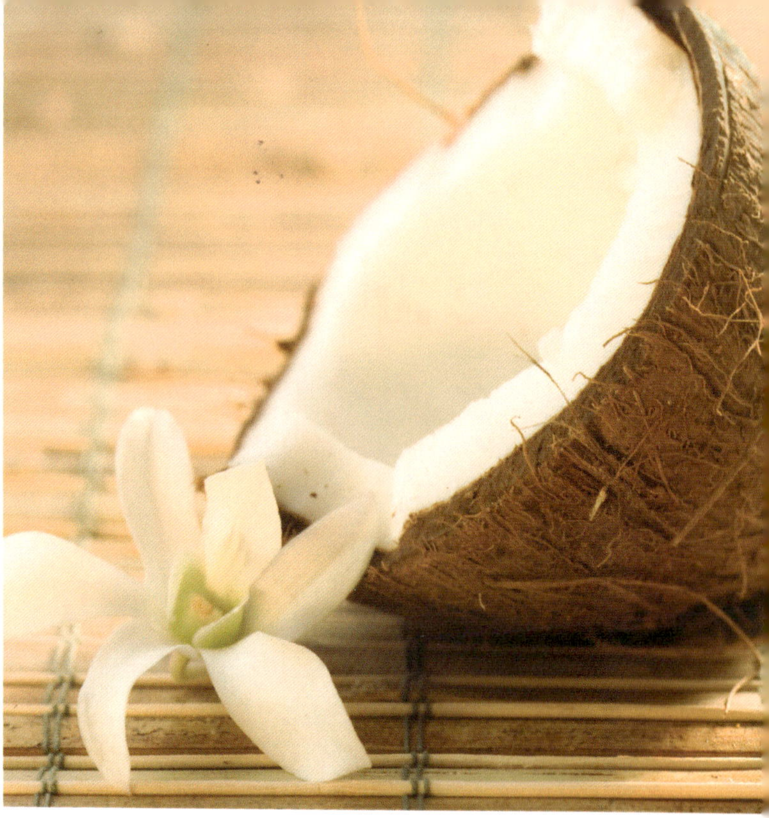

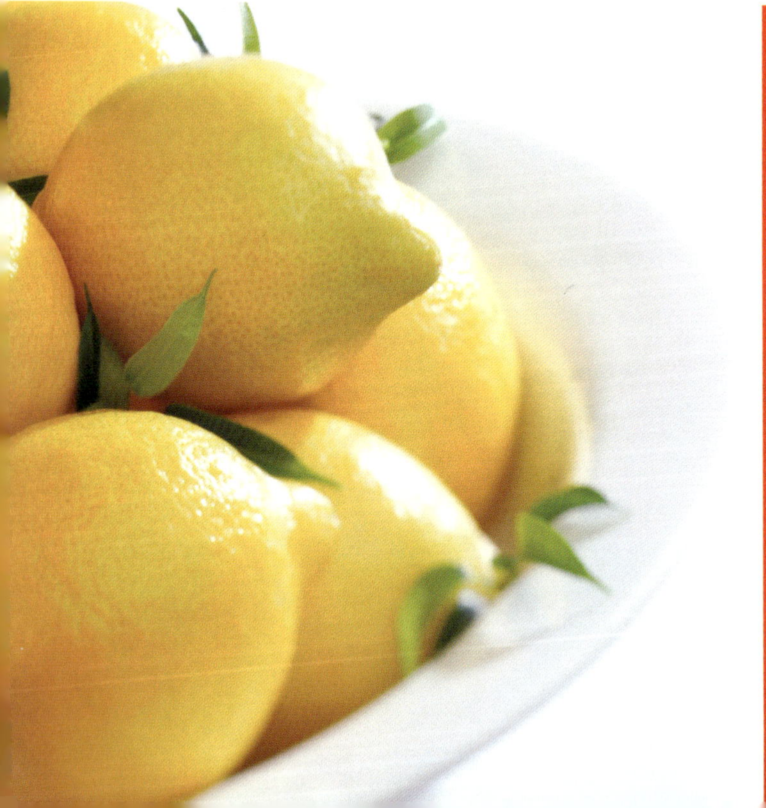

CONTENTS

Contents cont.

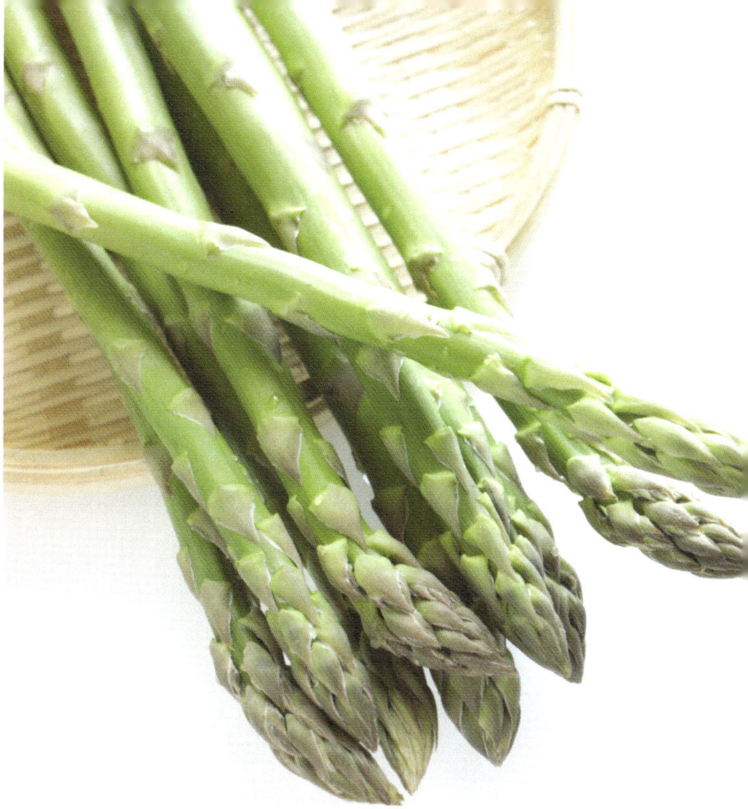

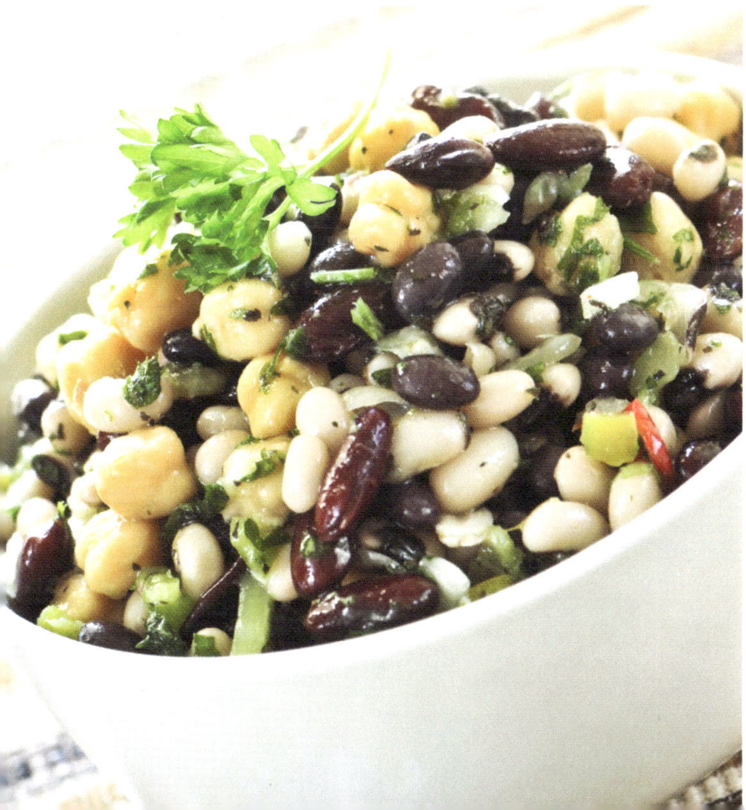

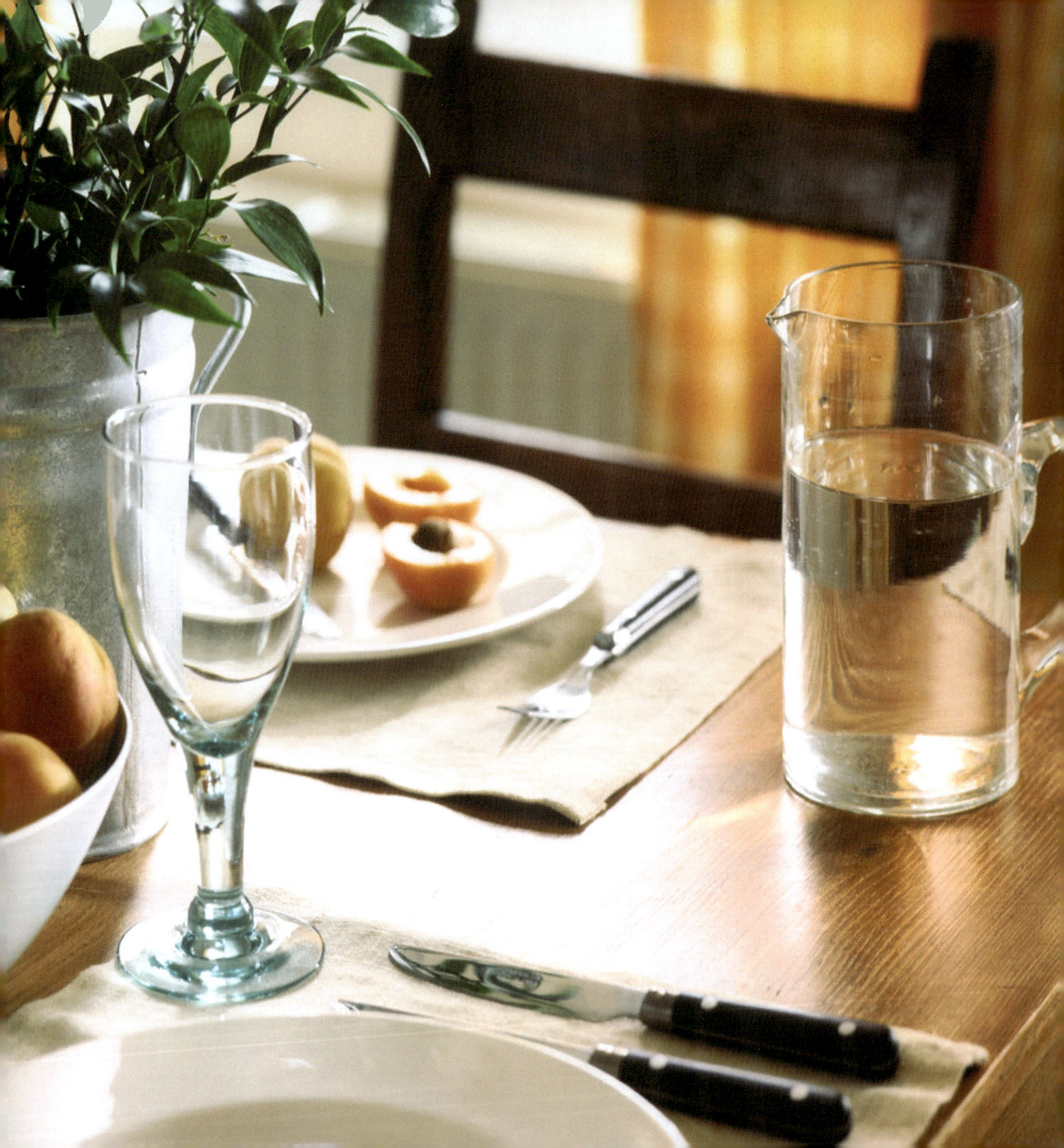

ACKNOWLEDGEMENTS!

I would like to begin by thanking God for preparing me to design and develop this cookbook. When I began the project, I did not have confidence in myself because I'm not a classically trained chef. However, through my quiet time with God, He showed me how to overcome my fears and realize the true blessing and gift that He has equipped me with to share with the world. The recipes in this cookbook were given to me by God, as I had never cooked these items before I started on Daniel Fast. I am truly grateful!

I would like to thank my lovely wife, Mary, for always being my supporter, my encourager, and my love. Thank you for always standing by me and helping me live out my true dreams. When I would say, "I cannot go any further with this project" or "It needs to be postponed until next year," you would always say, "No, now is the time for us to trust God!" You kept me going and for that I want to say thank you. I appreciate your confidence in me.

I would like to thank my parents, Larry and Cecelia Johnson. Thank you for instilling in me two principles: (1) I can do all things through Christ and (2) nothing is too hard for God. Also, thank you for showing me how to cook at an early age. This book is the result of your guidance and support.

Thanks to my sister, Lisa Johnson, for her excellent legal advice, and for always giving me ideas about things I had not considered for this project. Thank you for always supporting me in my endeavors. I would also like to thank Brownstone Publications for believing in my dream and making it become a reality. Without you this blessing would have been lost. Thanks to my pastors, Bishop Larry & First Lady Desetra Taylor of Center for Hope Ministries. I want to thank you for listening to God's Words and birthing the season of possibilities for my family. This cookbook is truly a manifestation of your obedience to God's Word.

I would like to thank the rest of my family and friends for all your support and love. Whether it was your excitement over the project, taste testing recipes to make sure they were right, or just speaking a word into my life, you've all played a special part in the creation of this cookbook. I love you and I thank God that you are in my life.

In closing, I dedicate this book to the memory of my family members who have passed way. Thank you for your love and encouragement. I know you are looking down on me and saying, "Go Mike!" And for that, I present this book in your honor.

I MADE IT... SO CAN YOU!

Introduction

Cooking has been a part of my life for as long as I can remember. I come from a long line of great cooks, so it was hard to be in the house without picking up a skill or two. As a young kid I learned to prepare fried chicken, macaroni and cheese, collard greens, and sweet potato pie—you know, the meals African-Americans commonly refer to as *soul food*. As I got older, I realized that I truly enjoyed cooking, so I began to expand my culinary expertise to include more elaborate meals. And before I knew it, people began requesting my services as a private chef and for catered events. I thought, *Wow, this is great!* I was doing what I loved and people were enjoying the fruit of my talents. It couldn't possibly get much better than that, right? That's what I thought. But little did I know GOD had something greater in mind. He had a plan to use my culinary talents as a tool to bless others and to glorify Him. And it all began with a decision to fast!

In January 2011 my pastor, Bishop Larry Taylor, announced that the entire church would participate in a 21-day Daniel Fast, which would require us to refrain from eating meat, sugar, and bread. Now I must admit, I was stunned by his words. Prior to this, I had never fasted from food for one day, let alone 21 days. So successfully completing this challenge seemed next to impossible. The idea was a shock all together, and my culinary brain went into overload. *How could I prepare a delicious meal for my family with such ridiculous dietary restrictions?* I wondered. Since I was a kid, every meal consisted of meat, starch, and vegetables. The idea of not enjoying such delicacies for 21 days seemed unrealistic. But nevertheless, I was up for the challenge. I was intrigued about how this fast would not only draw me closer to God, but how it might introduce my wife and I to a healthier way of living. We were at a point in life where we needed something from God. Though fasting wasn't a discipline we'd normally engage in, we decided it was time to do something different. Together we committed to the period of fasting, and thus our journey began.

I would love to say everything went smoothly once we began our Daniel Fast, but truth be told our first trip to the grocery store was nothing short of ridiculous. If you've ever participated in the Daniel Fast, I'm sure you can relate. I had every kind of fruit and vegetable you could image in the cart. I traveled to three different stores searching for key ingredients for traditional recipes I commonly cook, only to realize some of the ingredients didn't fit within the new dietary restrictions. Needless to say, I became frustrated very quickly. I soon realized the key to successfully completing this fast was preparation. So I decided to regroup and start again. But this time, I focused on meals my family loved and looked for ways to add a twist to the recipe without losing its delicious taste. Once I started preparing meals, new ideas and recipes began to take form. I was creating enjoyable meals that utilized the full spectrum of fruits, vegetables, and seasonings—healthy foods that were delicious to eat and nurtures the body. What was initially considered impossible became possible. Not only did I successfully complete my Daniel Fast, I finished with a closer relationship with God and an idea in my heart: a Daniel Fast cookbook, which you are holding in your hands today.

In *Divine Creations: The Daniel Fast Experience,* you will find recipes for exciting dishes that will warm your soul and provide healthier food options for your family. You will also learn how to prepare enjoyable and filling meals that exclude meat and other processed foods. This is truly a new beginning for you and I believe that you will experience a spiritual renewal and physical restoration in your health during this time of fasting. I pray that these recipes will provide you with a stress-free process for eating during your Daniel Fast experience so you can fully focus on what GOD has for you in this season of your life.

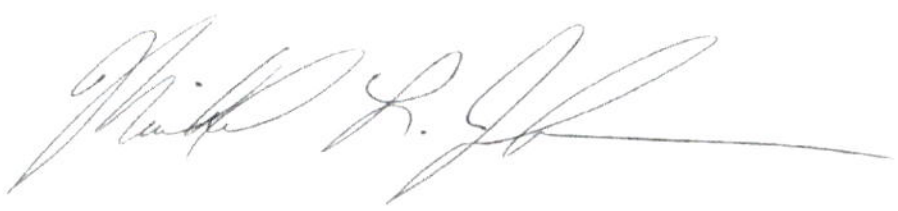

Michael L. Johnson

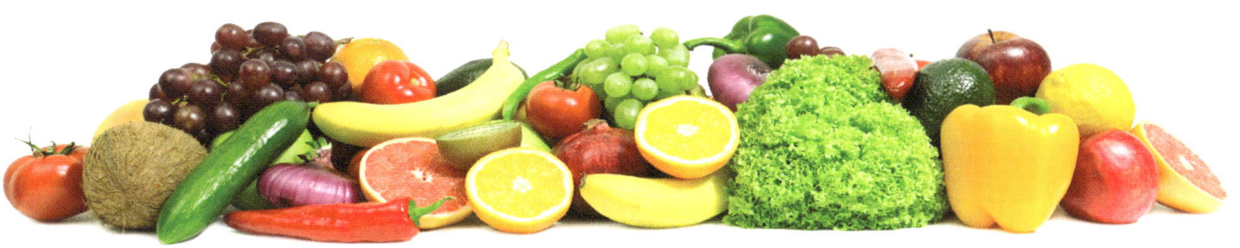

THE DANIEL FAST EXPERIENCE

Many people cringe at the idea of fasting for one day, let alone 21 days. And if you are anything like I was, the thought of abstaining from food for any extended period of time evokes a sense of fear of starvation even before the fast begins. If you think about it I'm sure you can remember a time or two when you worked yourself into a frenzy over what *could* happen while fasting. Thoughts like, "I'm going to feel sick." "I will be too weak to concentrate." Or my favorite, "What if I pass out from exhaustion?" Even as I am typing these statements, I can't help but chuckle at how funny we are when we are challenged to give up something that gratifies our flesh in any way. But through my own fasting experiences, I've learned that it's better to focus on what *will* happen instead of what *could* happen. For example, you will draw closer to God and purify your physical body. You will even learn how to exercise self-discipline. So there are many benefits to fasting. The more you are willing to sacrifice, the more God will release in your life. In this case, your sacrifice may be a favorite food, beverage or dessert. By denying fleshly desires, I believe you will receive more of God and more from God.

In saying this, I am in no way suggesting that fasting is an easy discipline. Like many of you I, too, enjoy a well-prepared steak with succulent, buttery potatoes. Or even a piece of fried chicken. But according to renowned author and speaker, Jentzen Franklin, the senior pastor of Free Chapel Church in Georgia, "Dethroning 'king stomach' is no easy task." However, it can be done. And when we stop listening to our flesh long enough to realize this fact, our perspective on fasting will change. The truth is I don't eat those types of food every day, and I would venture to say you don't either. So what are we really missing out on? It all comes down to this: we have to decide who is in control, God or the flesh? How much are you willing to give up in exchange for God's favor on your life? I was faced with this same decision a little over a year ago when I participated in my first Daniel Fast. Through this one decision, God blessed me with the vision to write this book. Through my Daniel Fast experience, God awakened a desire inside my heart and renewed my focus. I believe that you, too, can have an awakening of the desires in your heart. It will begin with fasting. Let's take a closer look at how the Daniel Fast can work in your life.

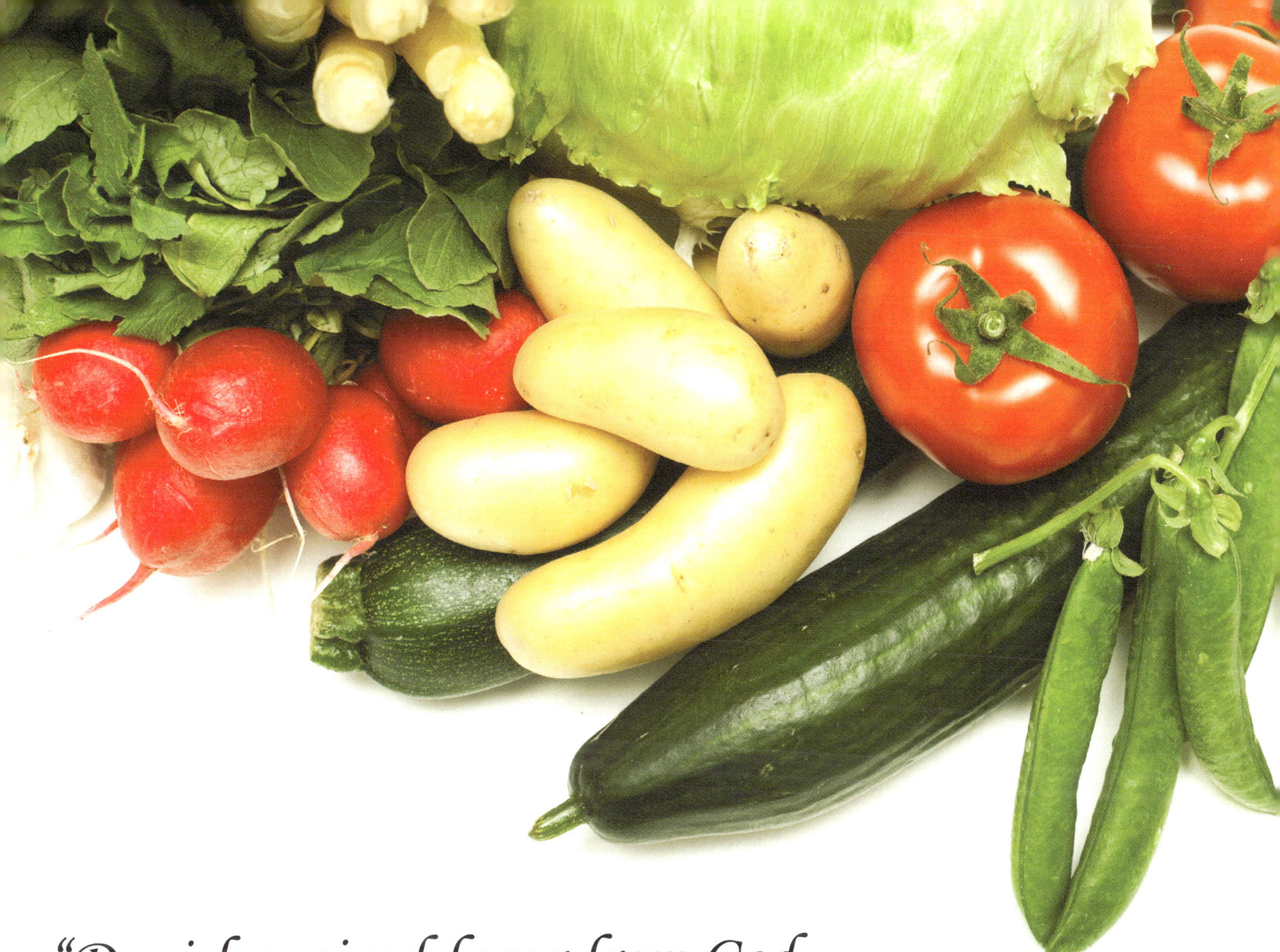

"Daniel received favor from God.

He increased in wisdom. He was more knowledgeable in visions and dreams. He even received an answer to prayer. Wouldn't you like to receive answers to prayers, increased wisdom, or the idea for business or book like I did? The answer is in fasting. Fasting can produce great things in our lives."

The Blessing of Daniel Fast

The foundation of the Daniel Fast is taken from the book of Daniel. This book records the life of Daniel, a Hebrew who was taken into captivity by the Babylonian army under the leadership of King Nebuchadnezzar. There are two occasions where Daniel committed to a time of fasting. The first is mentioned in Daniel 1, which states that Daniel declined the king's offer to partake in his choice food and delicacies. Instead of eating the King Nebuchadnezzar's meat and drinking his wine, Daniel asked if he could eat only vegetables and drink water for 10 days. As a result of Daniel's commitment, God blessed Daniel by giving him "knowledge and skill in all literature and wisdom" and "understanding in all visions and dreams" (Daniel 1:17). Daniel 10:3 records Daniel's second fast. Though it doesn't provide a specific food list, it does record Daniel saying, "I ate no pleasant food, no meat or wine came into my mouth, nor did I anoint myself at all, till three whole weeks were fulfilled." Again God blessed Daniel, but this time Daniel also received an answer to his prayer.

Look at the blessings that result from fasting. Daniel received favor from God. He increased in wisdom. He was more knowledgeable in visions and dreams. He even received an answer to prayer. Wouldn't you like to receive answers to prayers, increase your wisdom, or gain a new idea for a business or book like I did? The answer is in fasting. Fasting can produce great things in our lives. At first it appears that you are giving up a lot, but in the end you will gain so much. Daniel is our example of how fasting can produce powerful results. So, I encourage you to enter this time of fast with an expectation to receive something from God. Whether it's stronger faith, healing in your body, or renewed focus, there is a blessing for you in fasting. And as you commit to this Daniel Fast, avoid focusing on the do's and don'ts. I know there are differing ideas of what the Daniel Fast really is. People consume themselves with questions like, Can I drink 100% juice or does the fast require water only? Is it okay to have honey? Or what about herbal tea? Though these are valid questions, it takes our focus away from God and places it on food. In response to these questions, I would say this: the Daniel Fast is fruits and vegetables. What types and how they are prepared is a personal choice. Just remember why you are fasting – to draw closer to God, to purify your body, and to exercise discipline. Make this your primary focus, not what you can and cannot eat. I encourage you to seek God in prayer and allow the Holy Spirit to guide you during this time of fasting.

Preparing for Your Fast

You should never enter a fast without some level of preparation, both naturally and spiritually. Your flesh, or your desire for food, will at times be louder than your spirit. At some point it may seem your fast is not beneficial spiritually, as if you are hungry for no reason. But don't lose heart; fasting for any extended period of time can be intimidating. That is why it's important to make preparations for your fast. Here are a few tips to keep in mind:

Step 1— Have a Goal or Vision

Begin your fast with a clear goal in mind. Be specific. Why are you fasting? Is it for spiritual renewal, for guidance, or for healing? Having a vision will keep you focused during moments of weakness. Ask the Holy Spirit for guidance. Be sure to pray daily and read the Bible.

Step 2—Make a Commitment

Decide on the type and length of fast up front. Is the fast 10 days, 21 or even 40? Making a commitment ahead of time will help you remain focused throughout your fast, especially when temptations arise. Remember, use wisdom and prayer for guidance. If you choose to fast for extensive lengths of time you should consult your physician, especially if you have medical conditions.

Step 3—Prepare Yourself Spiritually

Though fasting has natural benefits, it's important to make spiritual preparations as well. In doing so, be sure to make prayer a daily priority, using your time of fasting to confess any sins, habits, behaviors, or areas of weakness that are not pleasing to God. Also, seek to forgive all who have offended you and ask forgiveness from those you may have offended. (Mark 11:25; Luke 11:4; 17:3-4)

Step 4—Prepare Yourself Physically

The Daniel Fast has natural benefits as well. In fact, it can cleanse the body and digestive system. In Dr. Don Colbert's book, *Toxic Relief Through Fasting,* he states, "Fasting is the safest and best way to heal the body from degenerative diseases caused by being overfed with the wrong nutrition."[1] So, fasting is a powerful tool and it's important to be physically prepared for the drastic changes that will result. Here are a few things to consider:

- Prepare your body. Eat smaller meals before starting a fast. Avoid high-fat and sugary foods.
- ***Medication should be withdrawn only with your physician's supervision!***
- Exercise moderately. Limit your activity. Spend time listening to praise and worship music. Read the Bible and pray as often as you can throughout the day.
- Take time to rest when you can.

When fasting, your body eliminates toxins from your system. This can cause mild discomforts such as headaches, leg cramps and irritability, especially during withdrawal from caffeine and sugars. Another side affect of fasting is hunger pains, periods of weakness, and tiredness. The first two to three days are generally the most difficult. As you continue, your body will adjust to the new physical changes. Remember to ***consult your physician before making any dietary changes, especially if you are on prescription medications***.

Step 5—Make the Most of Your Fast

Step one encouraged you to set a goal for the fast. But equally important is how you use your time during the fast. Be sure to set aside time for prayer and worship. You may even consider a schedule that outlines your day while fasting. This is important because it is easy to waste time, especially during moments of tiredness. You don't want to sleep your fast away. And when possible, avoid television or other distractions that will hinder your personal time with God. Remember, you are fasting for a reason, so make the most of your fast by planning your time with the Lord.

Step 6—End Your Fast Gradually

Once the fast is completed, begin eating gradually. Avoid overeating. Eat small portions, and slowly reintroduce foods to your digestive system. In *Divine Creations: The Daniel Fast Experience* cookbook, I have included recipes you can prepare once you have concluded your Daniel Fast experience. Check out the post Daniel Fast section in this cookbook for great recipes to help you in this transition process.

Fasting is a powerful discipline that can produce natural and spiritual results. The best way to ensure your success is through preparation.

As I bring this to a close, I want to encourage you to make the most of this time. Though this is a cookbook, remember that you are fasting. It's important to avoid being over consumed with what you can and cannot eat. Use this cookbook as a tool to help minimize any fear associated with fasting. The recipes are designed to alleviate your frustrations with dietary restrictions so that you can focus on what really matters the most – drawing closer to God. May God abundantly bless you while on your Daniel Fast Experience.

1. Colbert M.D., Don. *Toxic Relief: Restoring Health and Energy Through Fasting and Detoxification,* Florida: Siloam: A Strang Company, 2001.

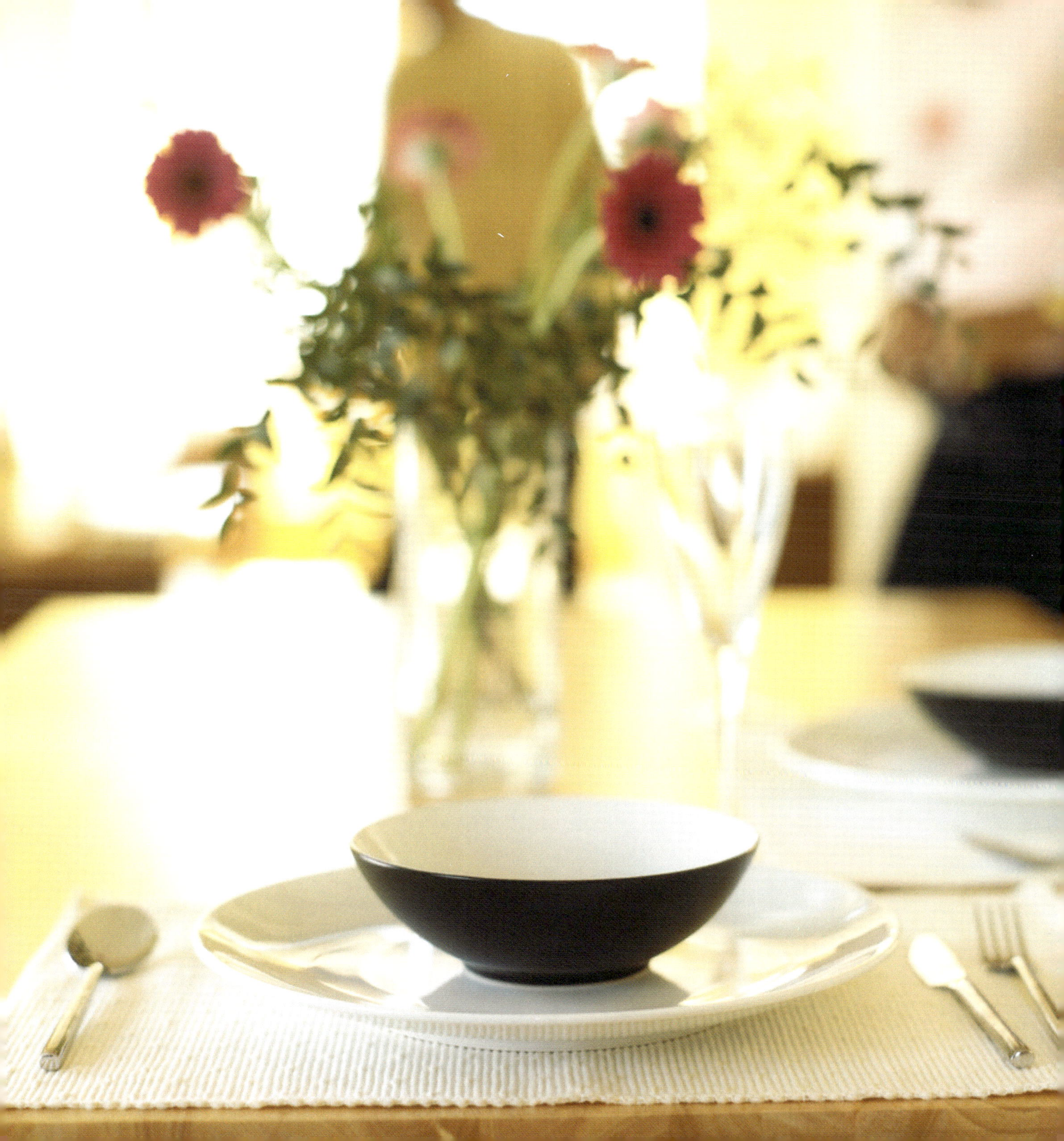

"Beloved, I pray that you may prosper in all things and be in health, just as your soul prospers." 3 John 1:2

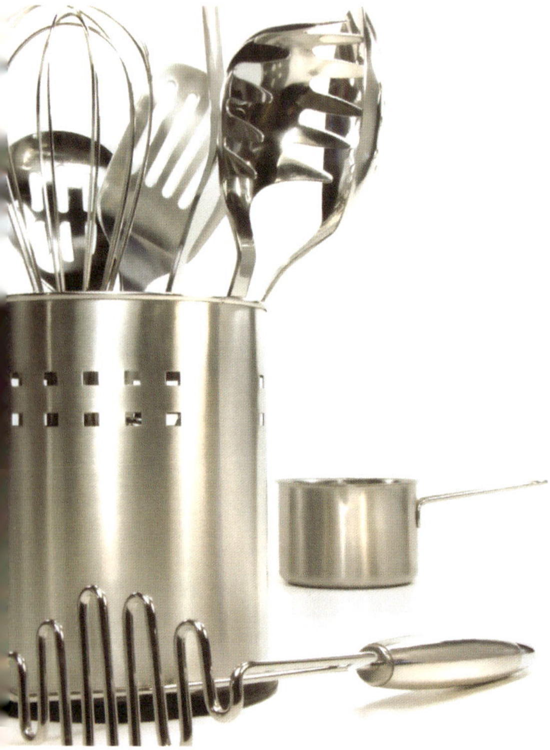

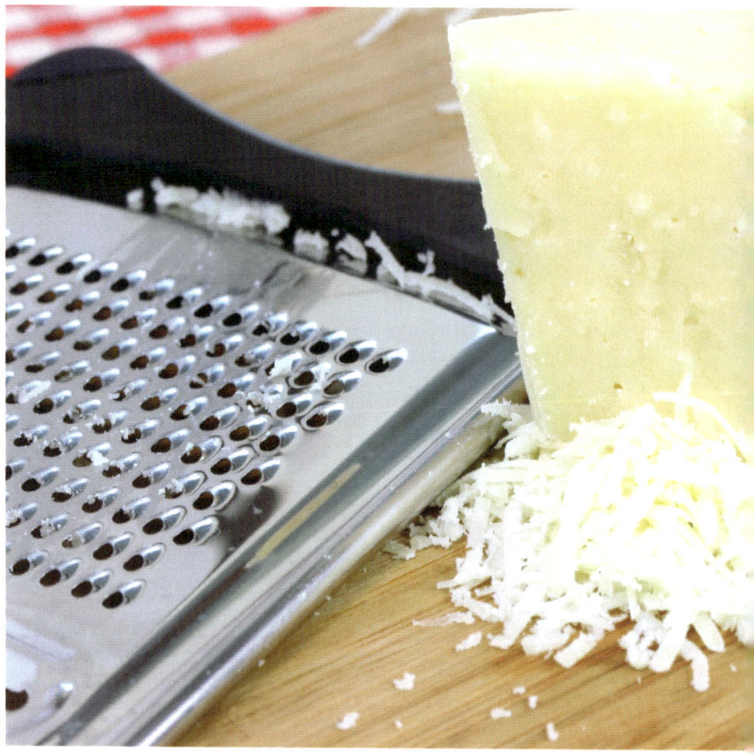

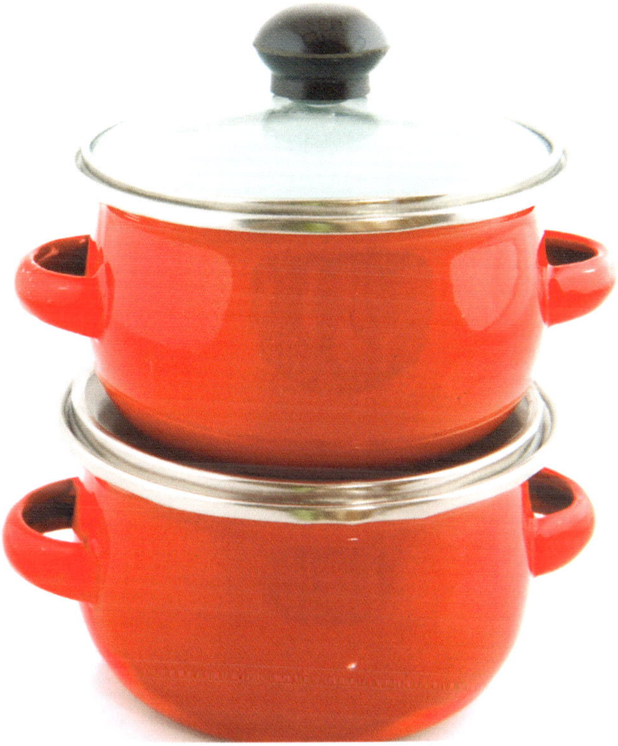

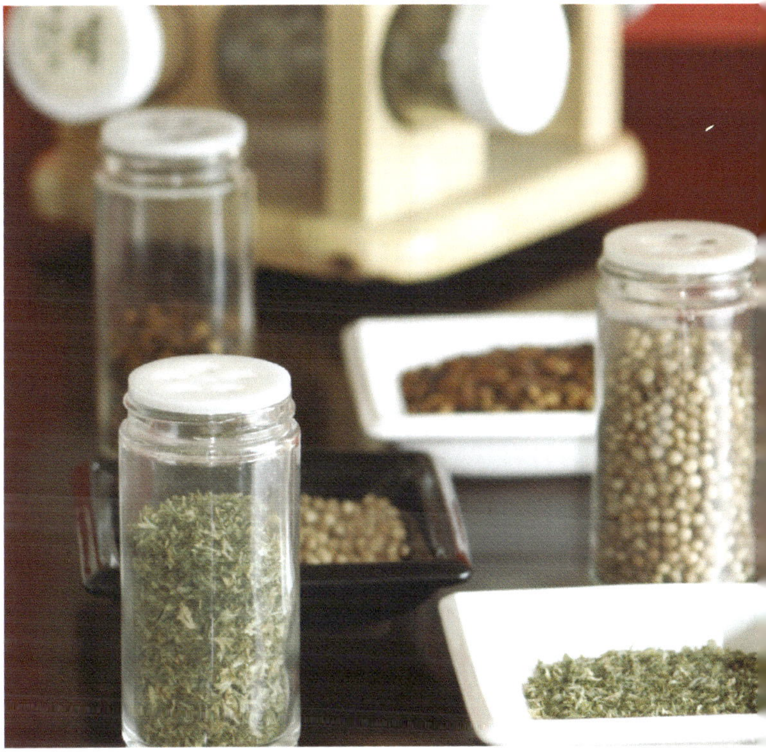

Kitchen Essentials

Fasting to Be Seen by God!

Matthew 6:16-18 NLT

And when you fast, don't make it obvious, as the hypocrites do, for they try to look miserable and disheveled so people will admire them for their fasting. I tell you the truth, that is the only reward they will ever get. But when you fast, comb your hair and wash your face. Then no one will notice that you are fasting, except your Father, who knows what you do in private. And your Father, who sees everything, will reward you.

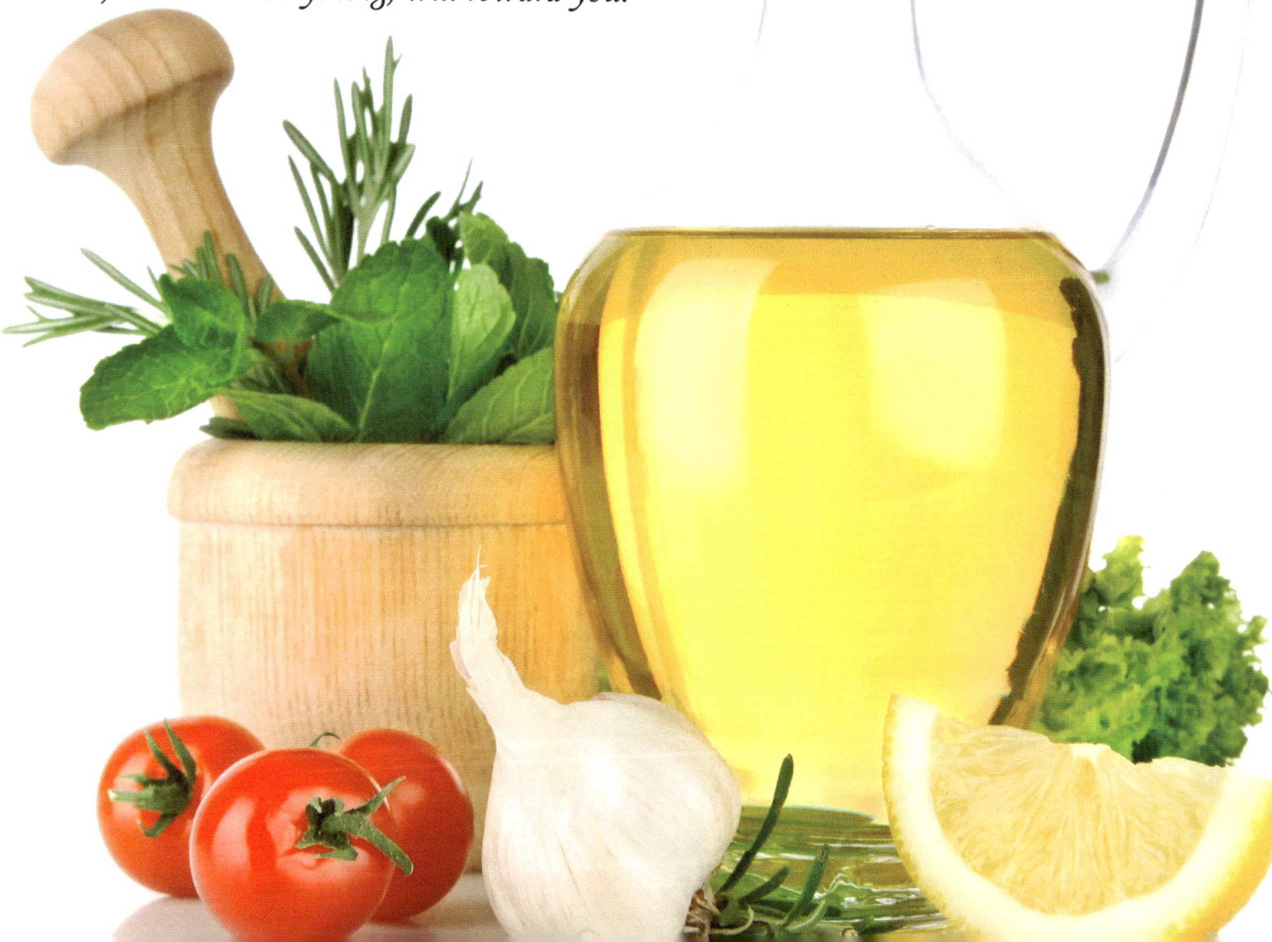

First Things First...Get Organized!

When you think of fasting, meal preparation is typically the furthest thing from your mind. However, with the Daniel Fast you are encouraged to enjoy choice delicacies like fruits and vegetables. But don't get too excited just yet! Having choices can sometimes cause frustration, and the last thing you want to do during your fast is become frustrated. So, I propose that you take a few days prior to beginning your fast to get things in order. Making time to organize your kitchen can help alleviate anxiety during your fasting experience. Here are a few tips to help you get started:

1. **Get Rid of Temptations.** Organize your pantry by removing foods you cannot eat during the fast. You don't have to throw food in the trash; however, it's a good idea to store items in a place where they won't be noticed. This will help avoid temptations during the fast.
2. **Determine Your Meals.** Creating a menu for the week is a great way to save time and money, especially if you are preparing meals for a large family. Planning a weekly menu makes you aware of your daily meals, and when followed it can help keep foods from spoiling.
3. **Shop for the Right Food.** Once you have created a menu, now it's time to go shopping. Create a shopping list for the week, using your menu as a guide. Also, when planning a meal, make sure you have the appropriate kitchen gadgets handy.
4. **Store Food for Later.** If you are extremely busy during the week, try using a Saturday morning or Sunday evening to prepare a few meals for the week, and store them in the freezer. Having precooked meals available will shave time from nightly dinner preparation. This will also help you avoid making choices that may compromise your fast.

By planning ahead, you will avoid wasting money and time running back and forth to stores—time you could use for prayer and devotion. Being organized will also ensure that your time is focused on God. Remember, your fast is about drawing closer to God.

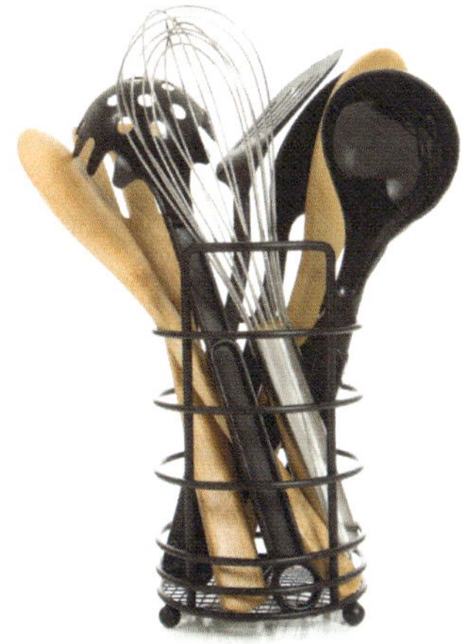

Cooking Utensils

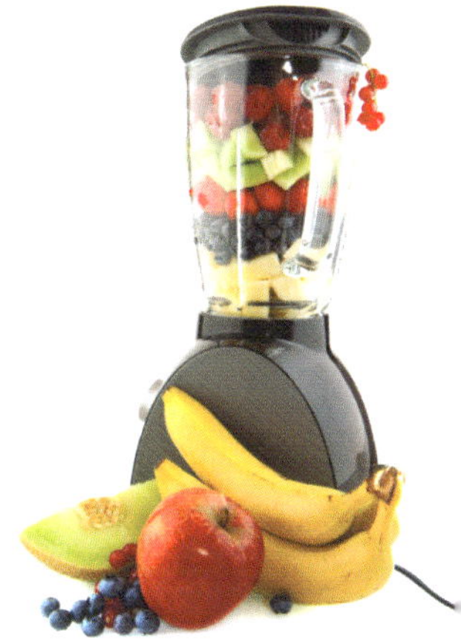

Blender

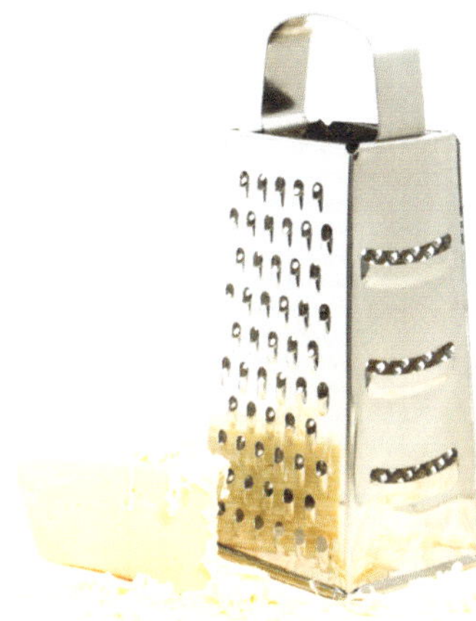

Grater

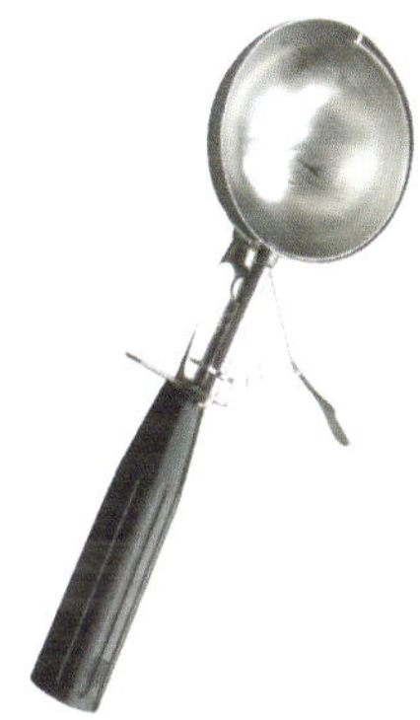

Ice Cream Scooper

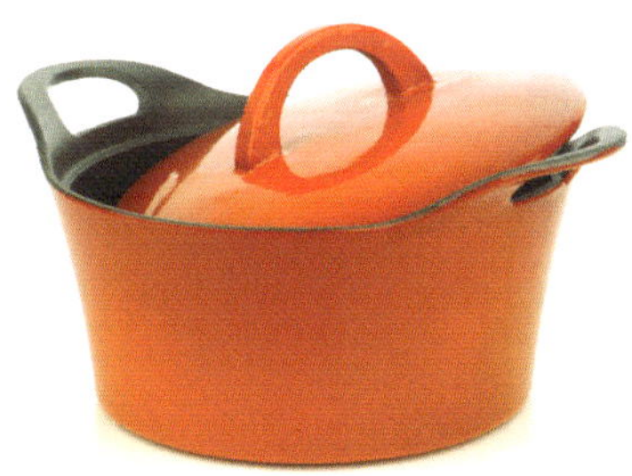

Heavy Stock Pot

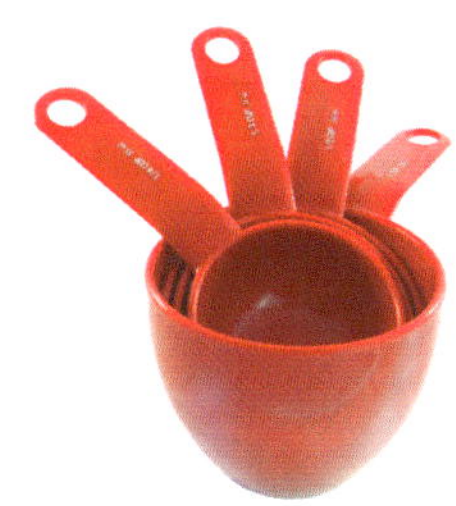

Measuring Cups

Adding Flavor to Your Fast

God loves variety! In fact, there are many natural herbs and spices available in a variety of shapes, colors and tastes for your enjoyment. Now, the key word is taste...flavor! These words are not usually mentioned when talking about fasting. But with the Daniel Fast, you can use a few natural herbs and spices to awaken your taste buds *without* compromising your fast. Herbs and spices like cinnamon, basil, garlic powder, rosemary, and oregano can add a lot of flavor to your fasting experience.

Common herbs and spices recommended for your kitchen:

- Cinnamon
- Chili Powder
- Thyme Leaves
- Cilantro
- Basil
- Black Pepper
- Pumpkin Spice
- Cinnamon Sticks
- Parsley
- Mint Leaves
- Cumin
- Garlic Powder
- Italian Seasoning
- Kosher Salt
- Onion Powder
- Nutmeg
- Ginger
- Cloves

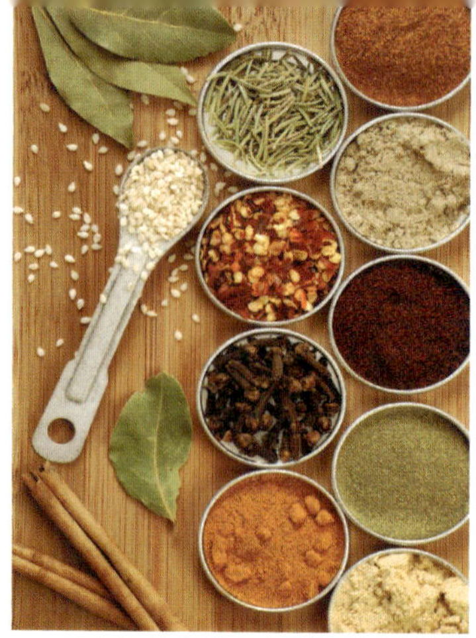

Seasoning Blends & Spices

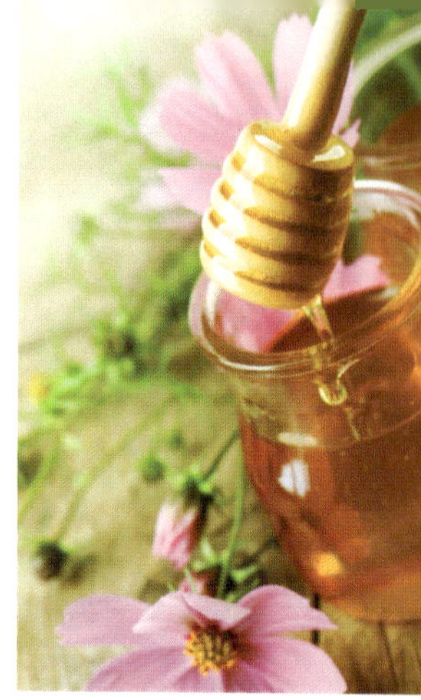

Natural Honey

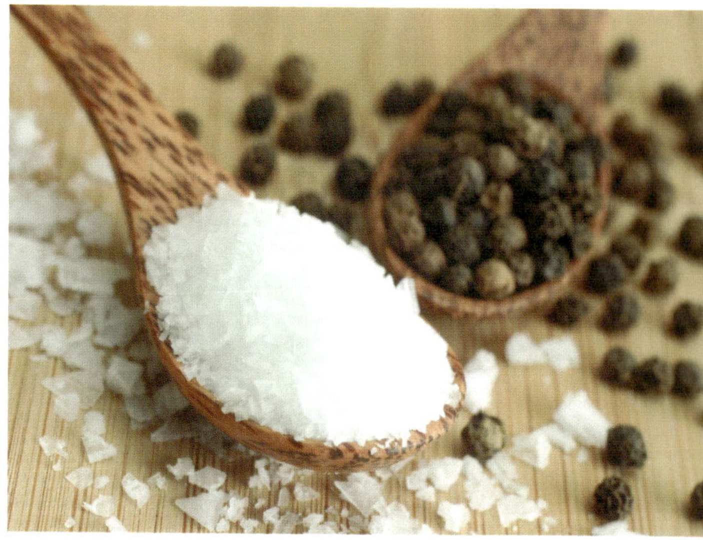

Kosher Salt & Black Pepper

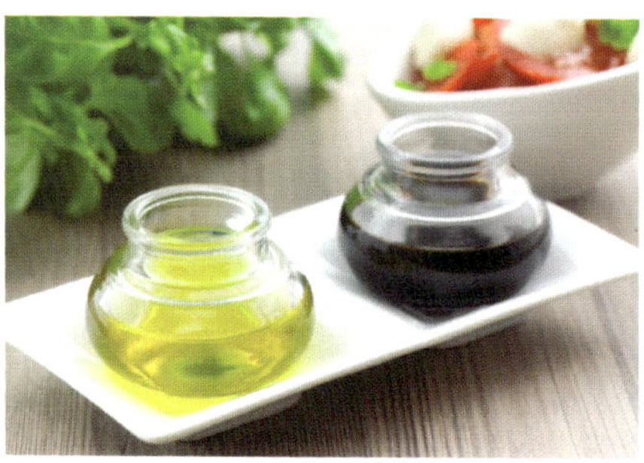

Oil & Balsamic Vinegar

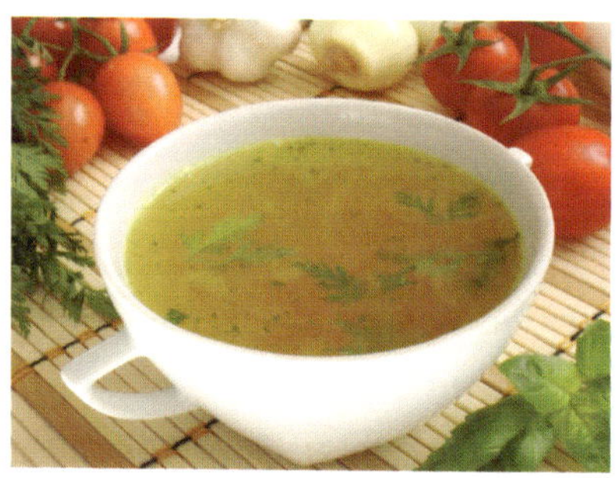

Vegetable Broth

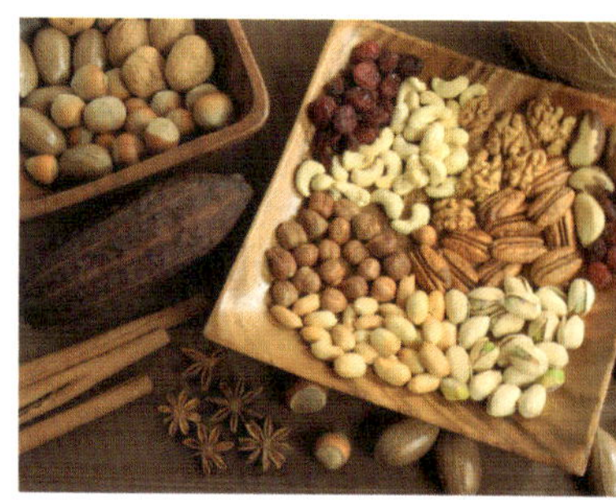

Assorted Nuts

God's Chosen Fast

Isaiah 58:6-9

"Is this not the fast that I have chosen: To loose the
onds of wickedness, to undo the heavy burdens, to let
he oppressed go free, and that you break every yoke?

s it not to share your bread with the hungry, and that
you bring to your house the poor who are cast out;
when you see the naked, that you cover him, and not
hide yourself from your own flesh?

hen your light shall break forth like the morning, your
healing shall spring forth speedily, and your
righteousness shall go before you; the glory of the
LORD shall be your rear guard.

Then you shall call, and the LORD will answer; you
shall cry, and He will say, 'Here I am.'"

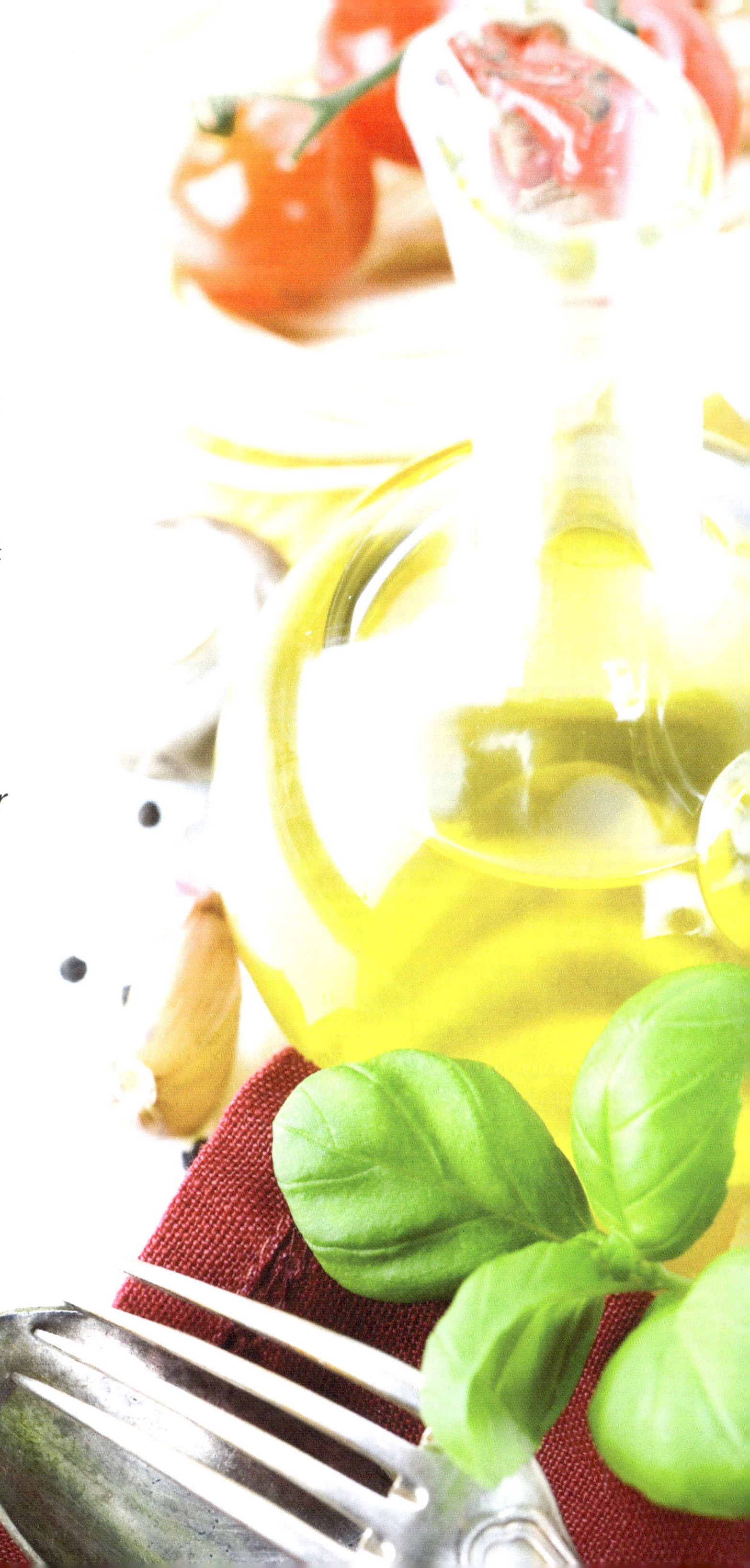

For I am about to do something new. See, I have already begun! Do you not see it? I will make a pathway through the wilderness. I will create rivers in the dry wasteland. Isaiah 43:19 NLT

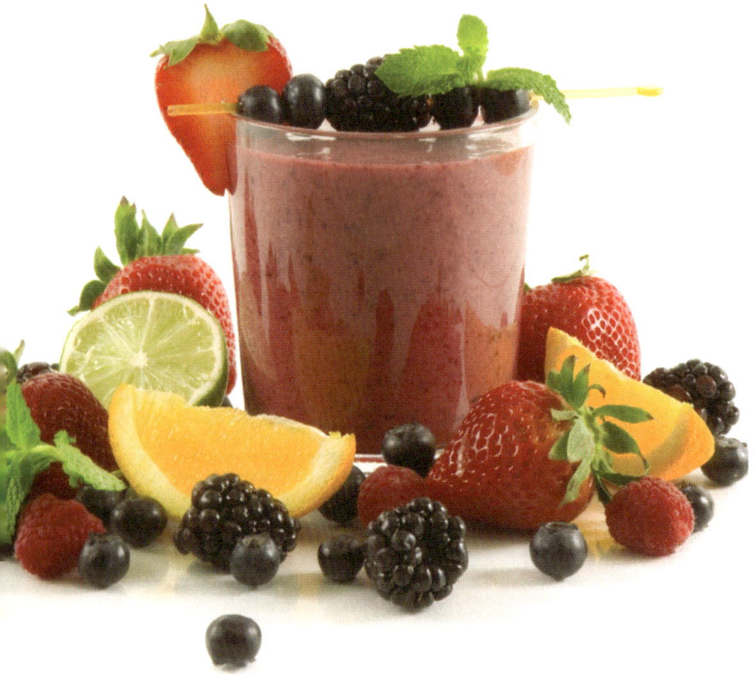

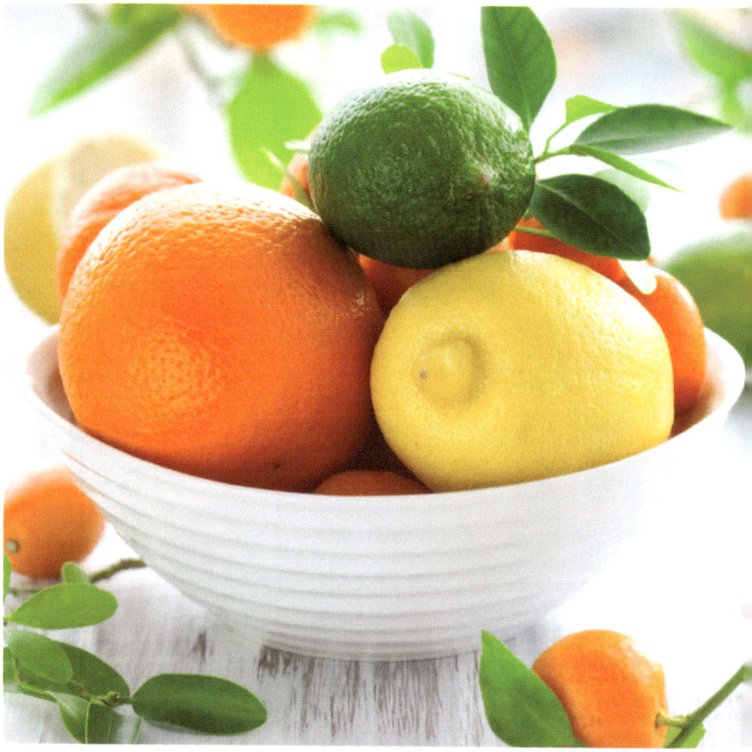

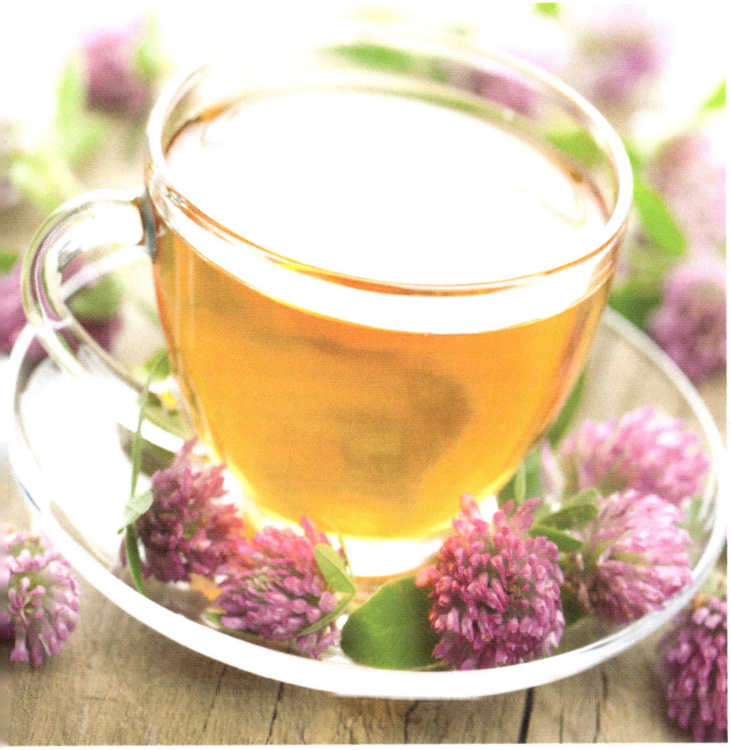

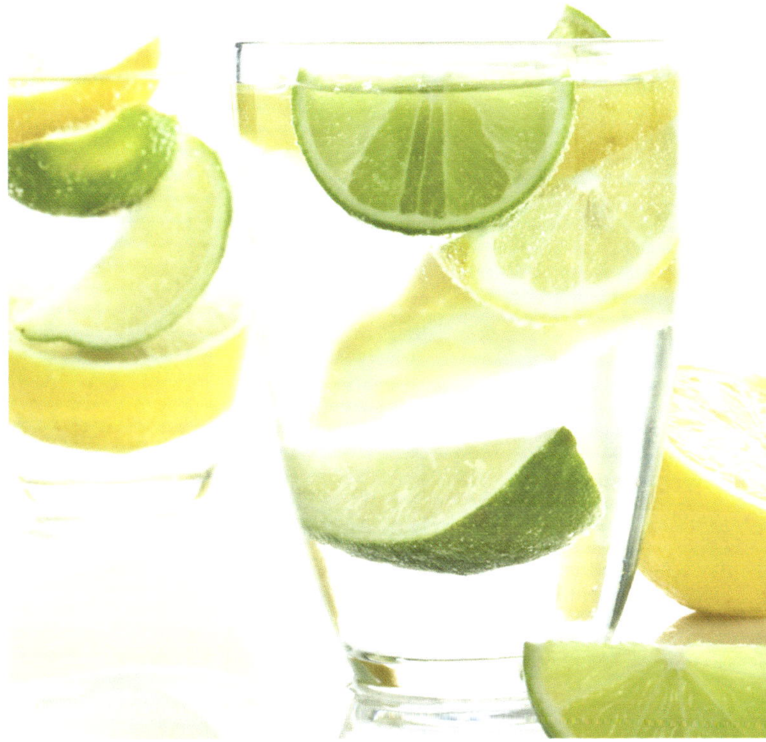

Beverages

Hot Apple Cider

8 oz. 100% apple juice

1 cinnamon stick

¼ tsp. ground cinnamon

Instructions

In a medium saucepan, combine ground cinnamon and apple juice. Warm over medium-high heat until bubbles form around the edge of the pan. Turn heat off and allow mixture to cool for 1 minute. Pour liquid into a coffee cup and add cinnamon stick for garnish.

Tip: This beverage can be used to replace coffee or tea cravings during the fast, as it provides your body with warmth.

Serving Size: 1

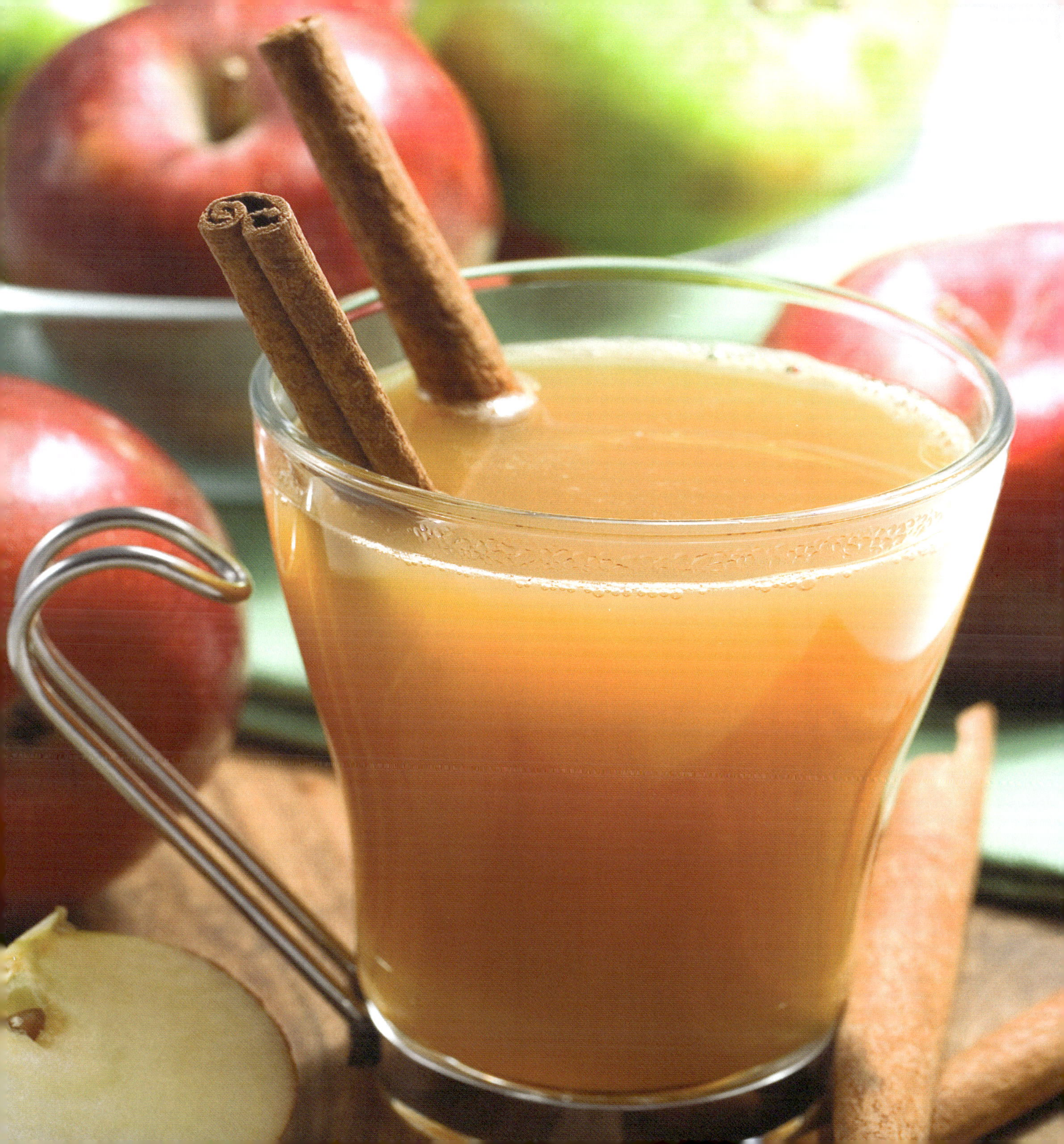

Lemon Infused Water

3 lemons, thinly sliced

1 cup ice cubes

5 cups distilled water

Instructions

In a 2-quart pitcher combine lemons, ice, and water. Refrigerate for 2 hours or overnight to allow the lemon to infuse water. Serve over additional ice cubes.

Tip: If you want a more intensely flavored beverage, add 2 sprigs of fresh mint or rosemary.

Serving Size: 5

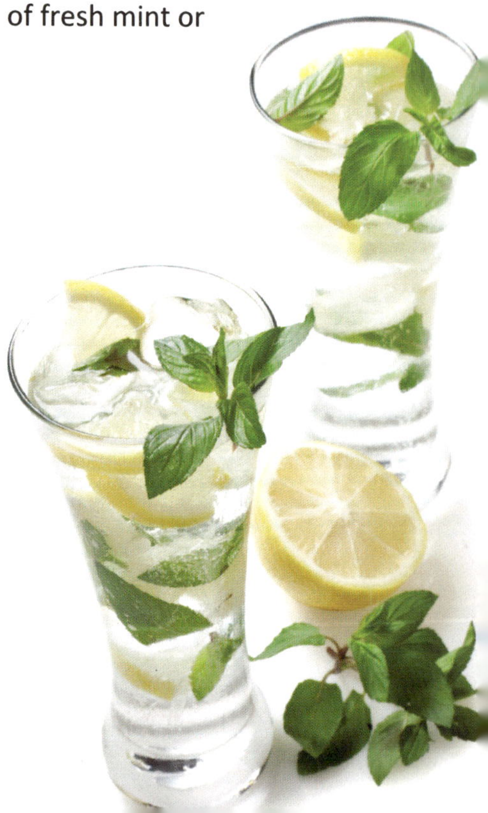

Lemon Mint Tea

1 sprig mint leaves

1 Celestial Seasonings® Lemon Zinger Tea bag

1 lemon wedge

1 cup boiling water

Instructions

In a medium stockpot bring water to a boil. Remove from heat and add tea bag to boiling water. Cover pot and allow liquid to steep for 5 minutes. Remove tea bag and pour lemon tea into cup.

Tip: Garnish with lemon wedge and mint leaf.

Serving Size: 1

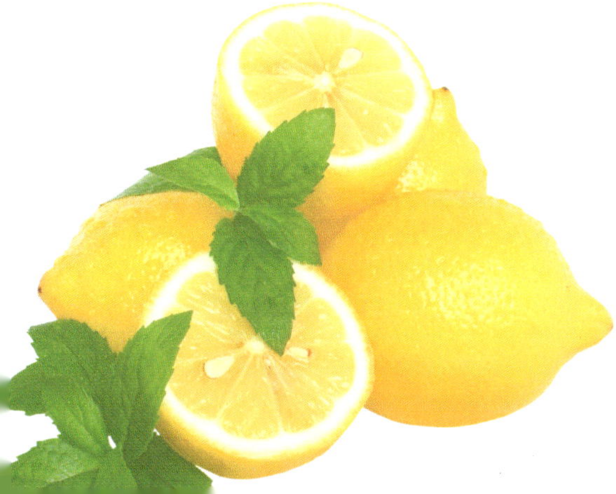

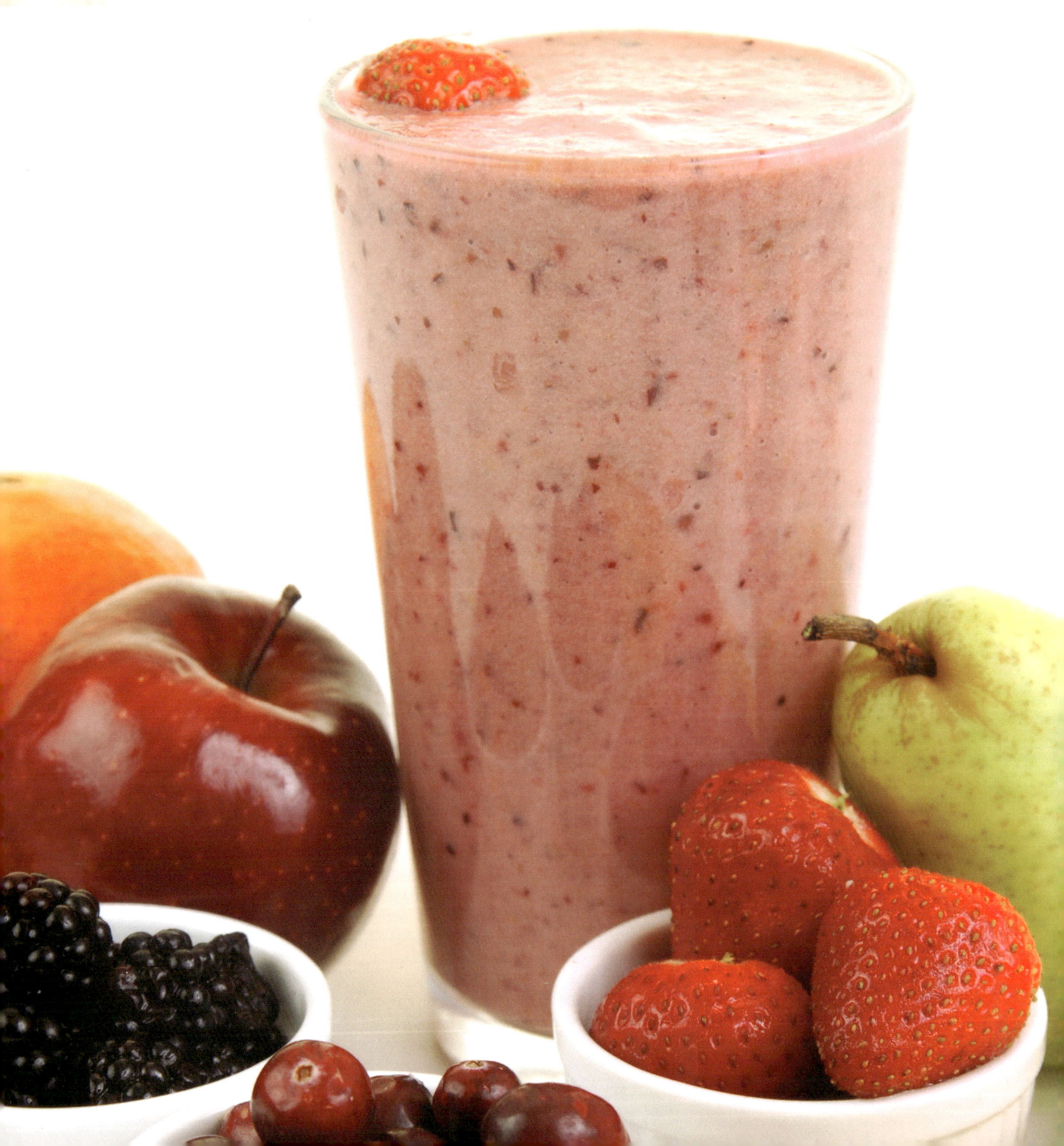

Fruit Smoothie

1 banana, peeled

8 oz. orange juice and/or apple juice

1 cup ice cubes

½ cup fresh blueberries

1 cup fresh or frozen strawberries

Instructions

Place strawberries, bananas, blueberries, juice and ice in blender. Use the ice crush setting to blend the mixture until smooth. If the texture is too thick, add an additional ¼ cup of juice. If it is too thin, add an additional ½ cup of ice cubes.

Tip: You may substitute any of the following fruits to create a different fruit smoothie: papaya, apples, blackberries, mango, watermelon, or kiwi.

Serving Size: 4

If my people, who are called by my name, will humble themselves and pray and seek my face and turn from their wicked ways, then I will hear from heaven, and I will forgive their sin and will heal their land. 2 Chronicles 7:14 NIV

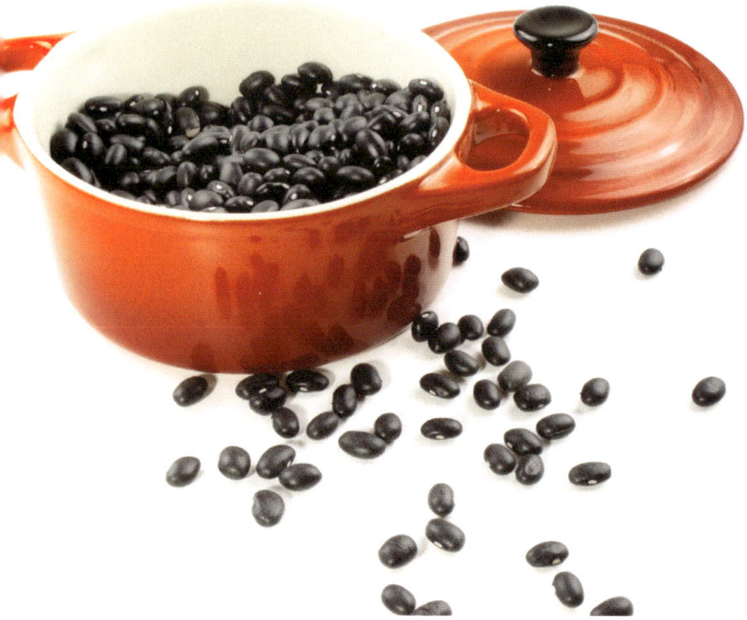

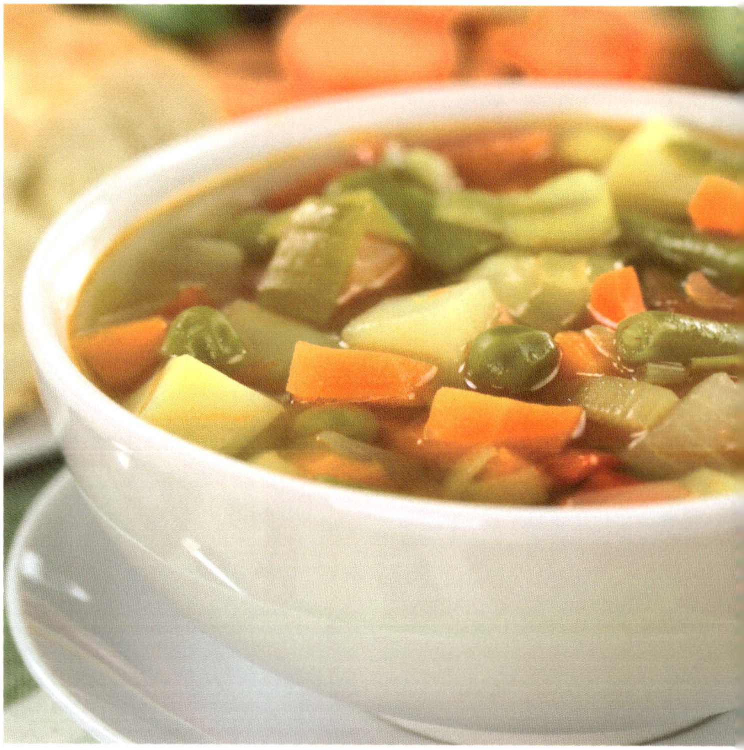

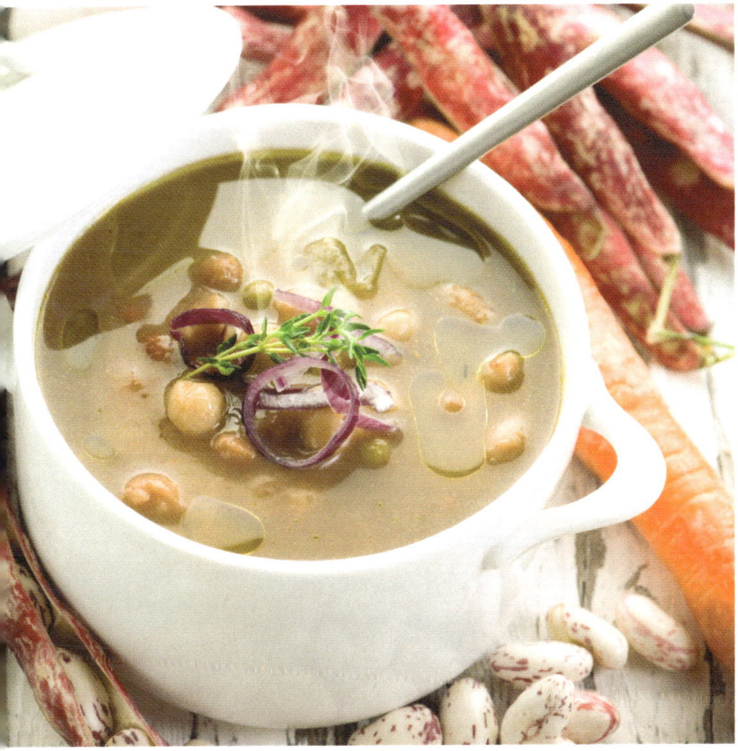

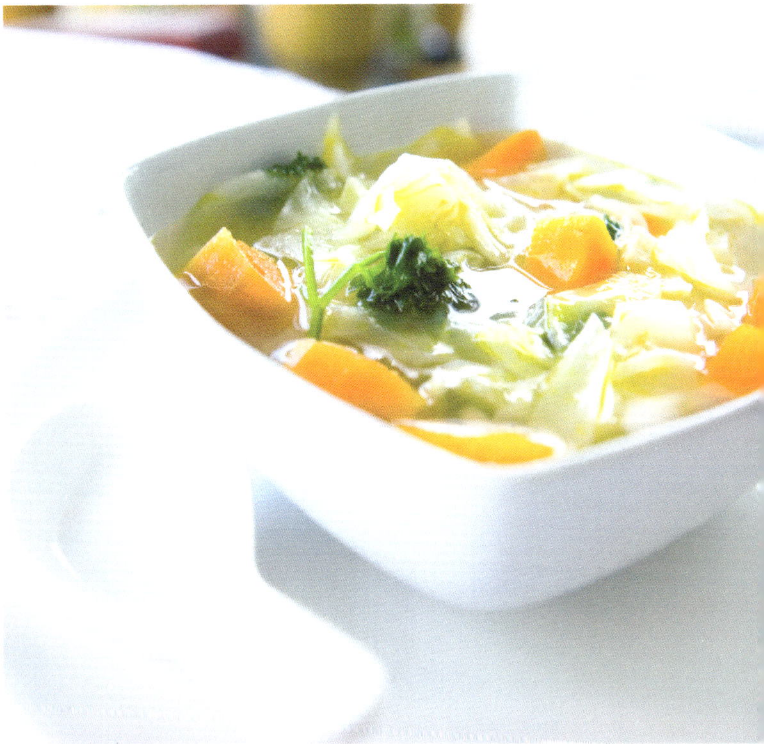

Soups

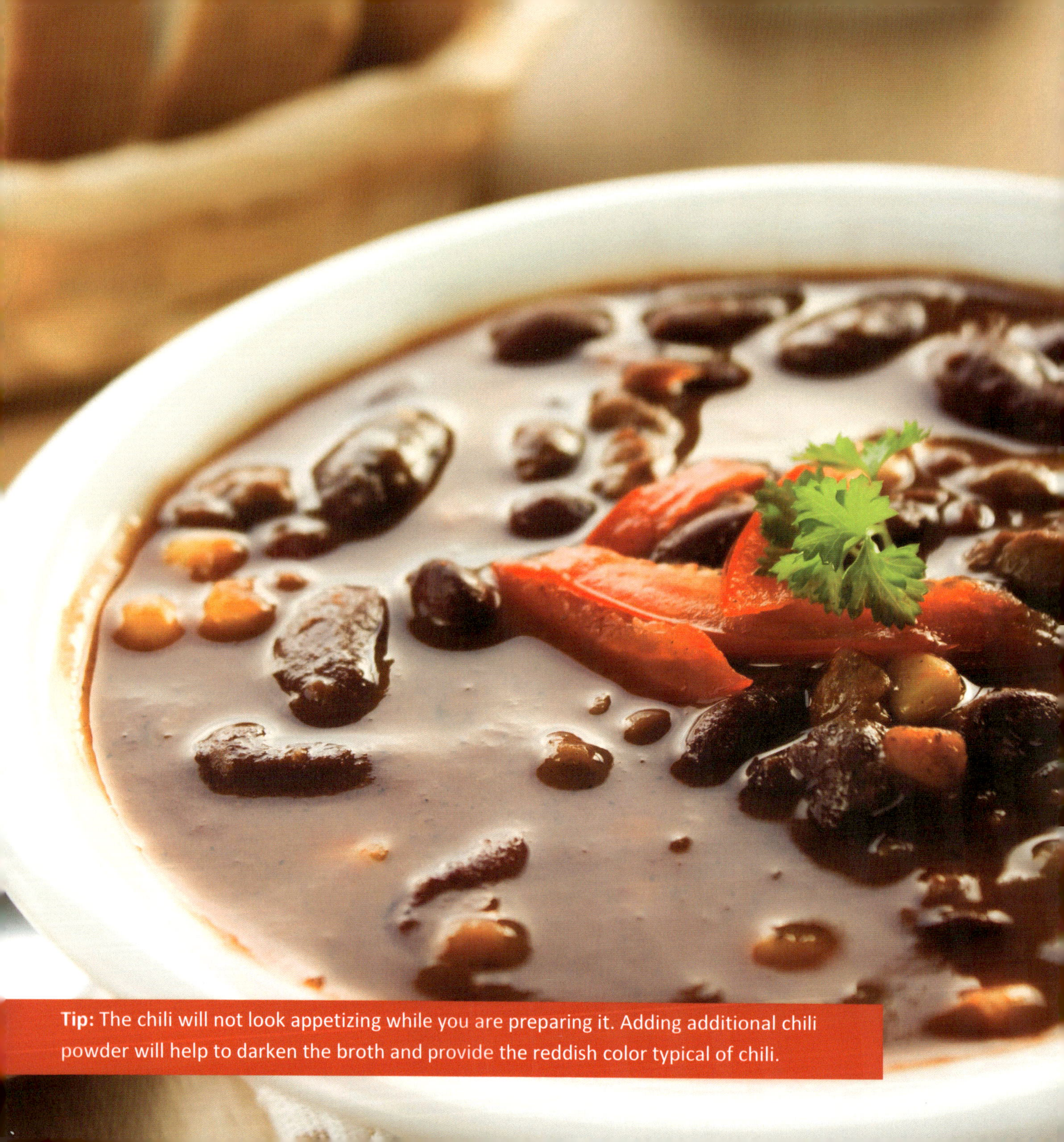

Tip: The chili will not look appetizing while you are preparing it. Adding additional chili powder will help to darken the broth and provide the reddish color typical of chili.

Meatless Chili

2 tbs. olive oil

1 large onion, minced

1 green pepper, chopped

3 garlic cloves, minced

1 tsp. adobe seasoning

1 tsp. ground cumin

½ tsp. crushed red pepper flakes

4 cups water

1 large dollop of tofu sour cream

1 package Lifelight Smart Ground® Original Veggie Protein Crumbles

2 tbs. chili powder plus 1 tbs. additional chili powder

1 can Hunt's diced fire roasted tomatoes with garlic (14.5 oz.)

2 cans light red kidney beans, drained (16 oz.)

Instructions

In a large stockpot sauté onions and green pepper in olive oil until onions are translucent (about 10 minutes). Add garlic and cook for another 2 minutes. Add kidney beans, ground veggie protein crumbles, and tomatoes and stir. Add chili powder, cumin, red pepper flakes, and abode seasoning to mixture and stir. Add water and simmer uncovered on medium-high heat for 30-45 minutes. Stir occasionally to prevent burning. The chili will start to thicken while simmering. Add the remaining chili powder for additional color. Serve in a soup bowl and finish with a dollop of tofu sour cream (see page 46 for recipe).

Serving Size: 8

Potato Leek Soup

2 tbs. olive oil

1 onion, finely chopped

1 tsp. kosher salt

½ tsp. black pepper

1 green onion stalk, chopped

2 leeks, cleaned and cut into 1-inch pieces

2 russet potatoes, peeled and quartered

1 can vegetable broth (32 oz.) plus 1 cup cold water if needed

Instructions

Cut leeks length wise and clean them by running under cold water and separating each layer to remove sand. Cut dark green leaves off, and only use the white and light green portion of leeks. Cut leeks and onions as instructed above.

In a large stockpot add olive oil and heat to medium-high. Add onions to the olive oil and sauté 1-2 minutes, or until onions are translucent. Add the leeks and sauté until tender. Add salt and pepper. Remove from heat and prepare potatoes as instructed; add potatoes to the mixture and return pot to medium-high heat. Add vegetable broth and simmer for 30-45 minutes or until potatoes are tender. You may need to add additional water if the broth evaporates too quickly.

Once potatoes are tender, remove them from heat and allow the soup to cool for approximately 5 minutes. Transfer 1-2 ladles of soup to an electric blender. Blend

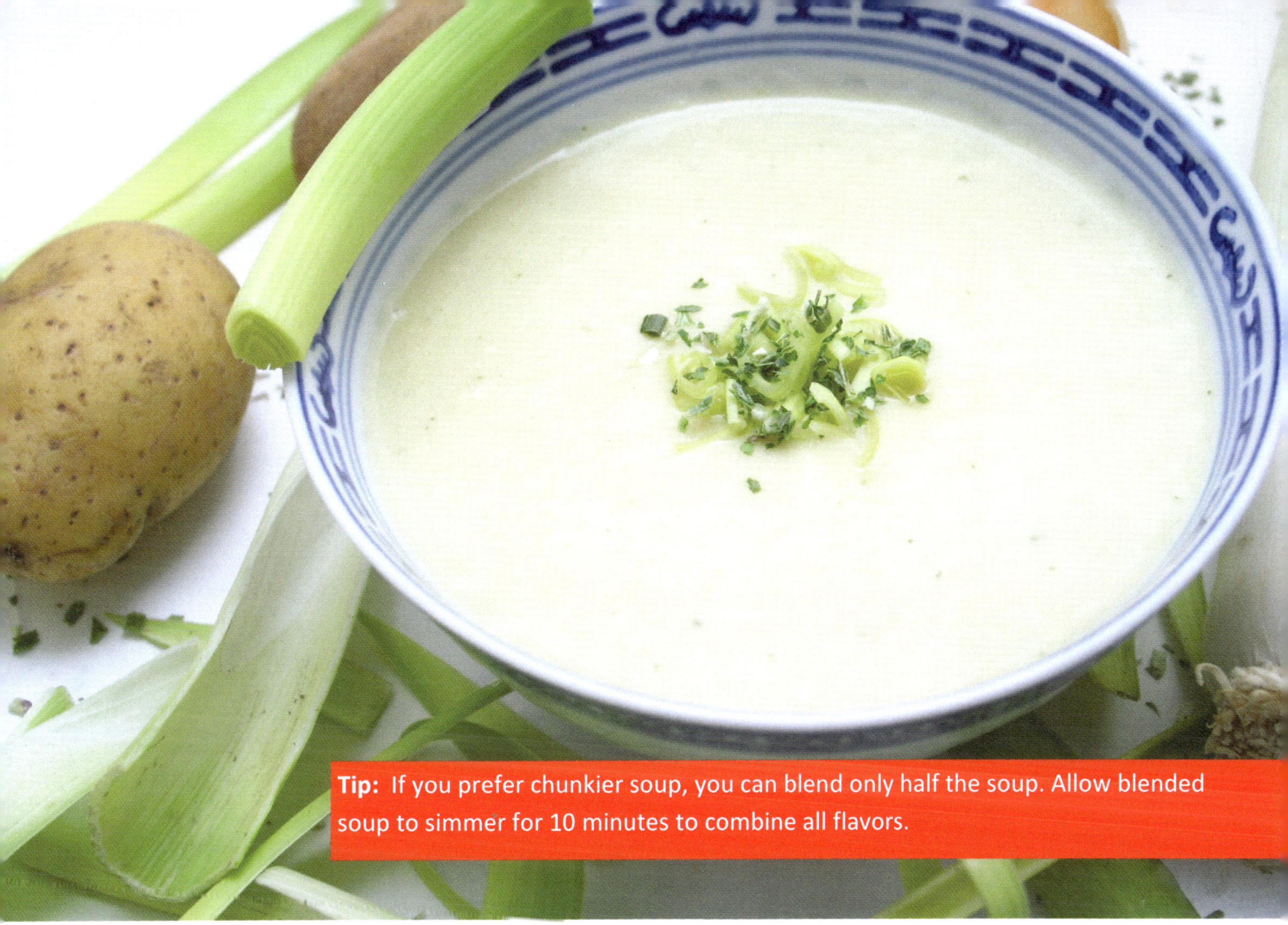

Tip: If you prefer chunkier soup, you can blend only half the soup. Allow blended soup to simmer for 10 minutes to combine all flavors.

soup in small batches on the liquefy setting, and pour blended soup into another stockpot. When complete adjust seasonings to suit your taste preference. Serve in a soup bowl and garnish with green onions.

Serving Size: 4

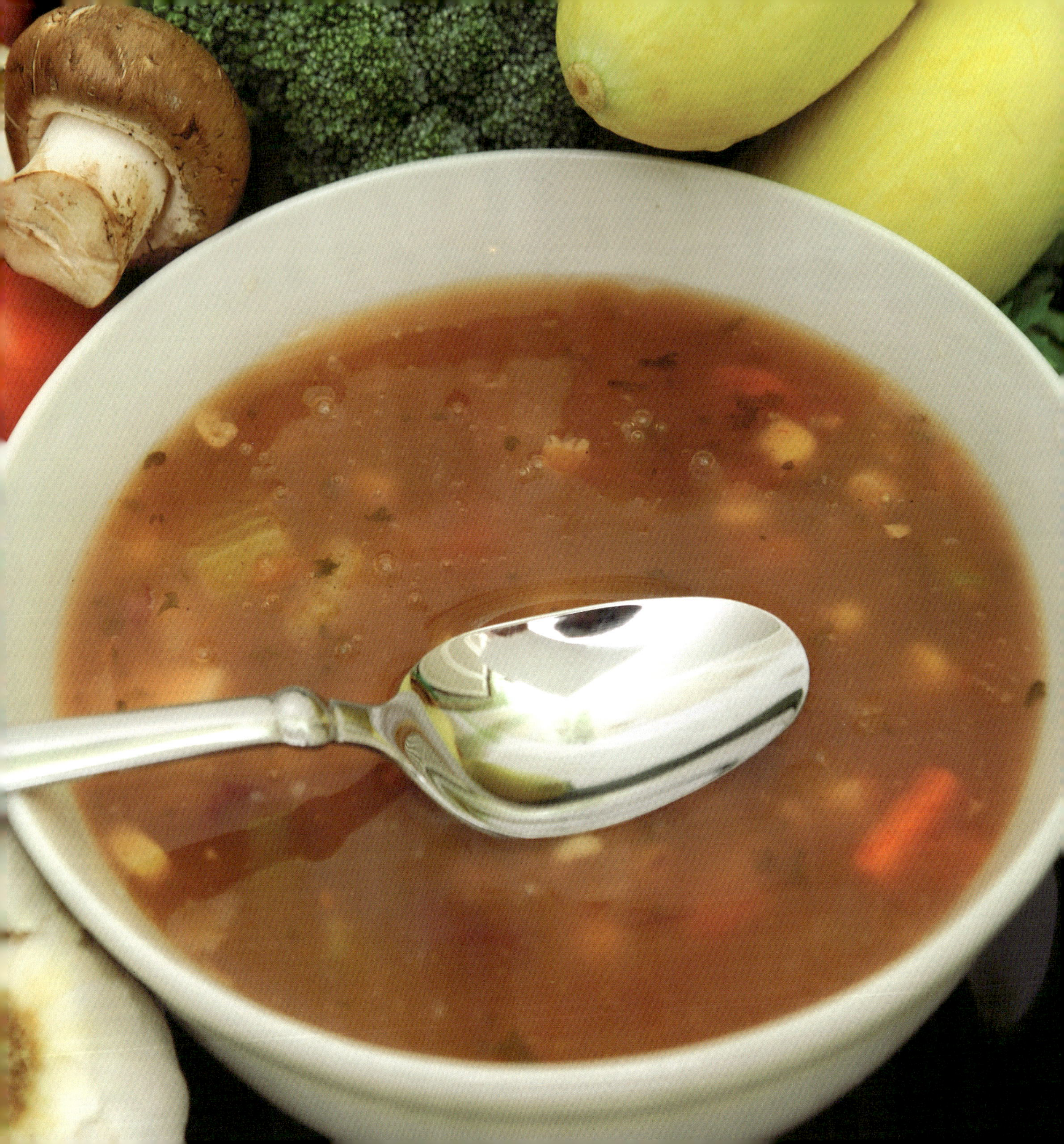

Vegetable Soup

3 large carrots, diced

1 large onion, diced

2 garlic cloves, minced

2 tsp. kosher salt

½ tsp. dried thyme leaves

1 tbs. tomato paste

½ lbs. fresh green beans

3 russet potatoes, peeled and quartered

3 celery stalks, diced

3 tbs. olive oil

½ tsp. black pepper

2 bay leaves

1 bag frozen corn

1 box vegetable broth (32 oz.)

3 cups water

Instructions

Prepare onion, celery, carrots, and potatoes as instructed. Sauté all vegetables in a large pot with olive oil for about 5 minutes. Add salt, pepper, garlic, and thyme to mixture and cook for an additional 1-2 minutes. Add vegetable broth and water. Include tomato paste and bay leaves to soup mixture and bring to a boil. Boil for 30 minutes on medium-high heat. Add green beans and frozen corn and allow the soup to simmer for an additional 20 minutes on low heat until green beans are tender.

Serving Size: 4

16 Bean Soup

3 large carrots, diced

1 large onion, diced

3 celery stalks, diced

1 large green bell pepper, minced

5 garlic cloves, minced

3 tbs. olive oil

2 tsp. kosher salt

½ tsp. black pepper

2 bay leaves

½ tsp. dried thyme leaves

1 tbs. tomato paste

2 cans vegetable broth (14 oz.)

3 cups water

½ lb. Goya 16 beans soup mix, prepared as instructed on package

Instructions

Prepare beans as instructed on package; overnight soak process is best. Be sure to remove any debris from the beans prior to preparing the soup.

In a large stockpot add olive oil and sauté onion, celery, carrots, green bell pepper, and garlic until vegetables are tender. Add salt, pepper, and thyme to mixture. Next, include prepared beans. Add vegetable broth and water. Include tomato paste and bay leaves and bring mixture to a boil. Simmer on medium to low heat until beans are tender.

Serving Size: 6

Tip: You may have to add additional water or vegetable broth because the beans will absorb the liquid as the soup simmers.

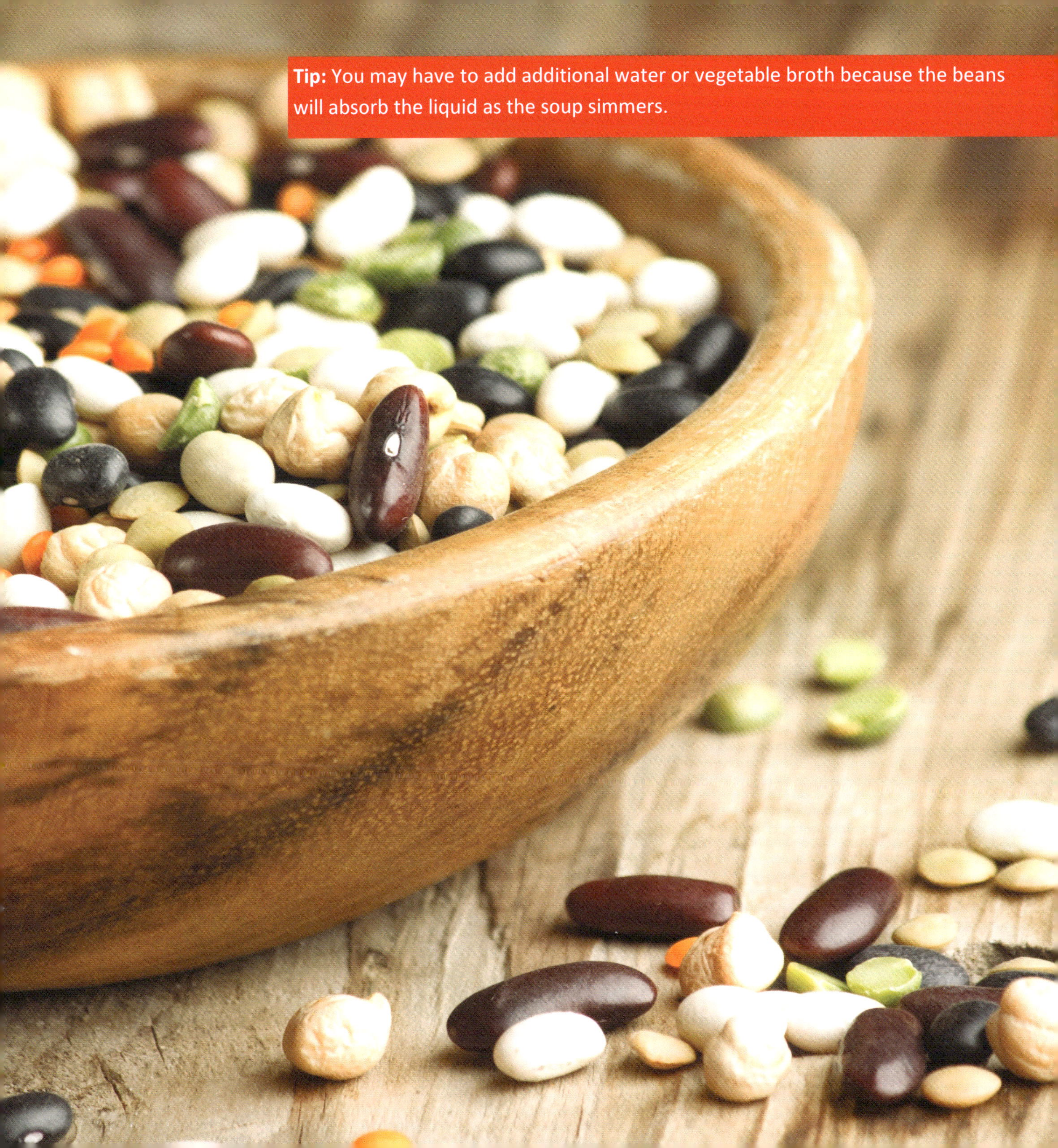

Black Bean Soup

3 tbs. olive oil

1 green bell pepper, diced

3 small carrots

¼ tsp. garlic powder

2 ½ tsp. kosher salt

1 bay leaf

4 cups vegetable broth

1 cup whole wheat brown rice, cooked

1 bag dried black beans

1 medium onion, diced

1 medium jalapeño, seeded and diced

1 tsp. cumin

½ tsp. black pepper

1 tsp. adobe seasoning

4 cups water

Instructions

Prepare dried black beans by allowing them to soak overnight in 2 cups of water. Be sure to remove any debris from the beans prior to preparing the soup.

In a large stockpot add olive oil and sauté bell pepper, onion, carrots, and jalapeños over medium-high heat until onions are translucent and soft. Add salt, black pepper, adobe seasoning, cumin, and garlic powder. Add 2 cups of the water and all of the vegetable broth. Bring the soup up to boil, add bay leaves, and adjust seasoning to taste. Simmer for 1½ hours until beans are soft. Add the additional 2 cups of water to pot as water starts to evaporate during the boiling process. Before serving, I recommend that you add 1 tablespoon of cooked whole wheat brown rice for additional texture.

Serving Size: 8

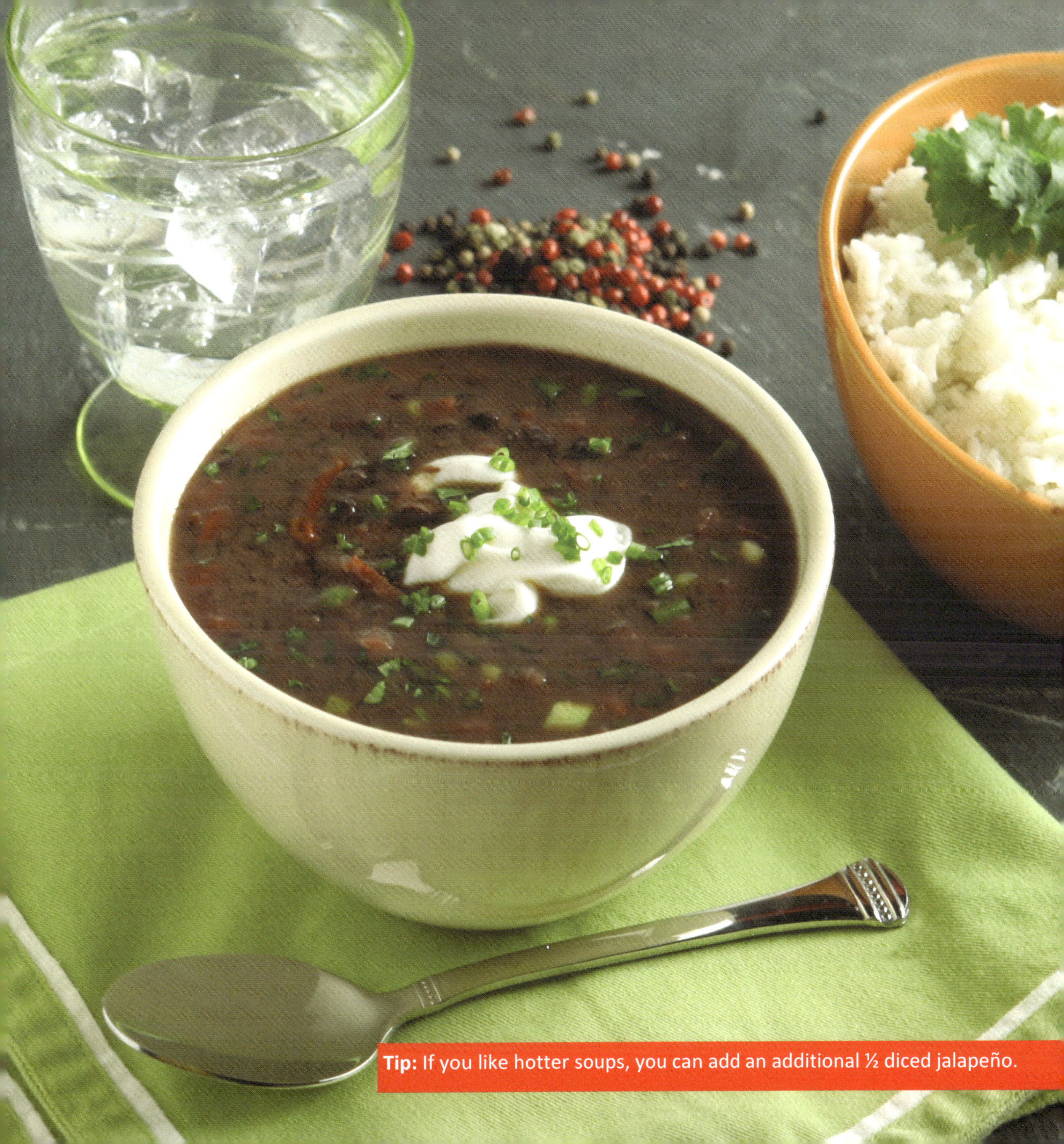

Tip: If you like hotter soups, you can add an additional ½ diced jalapeño.

And without faith it is impossible to please God, because anyone who comes to him must believe that he exists and that he rewards those who earnestly seek him. Hebrews 11:6 NIV

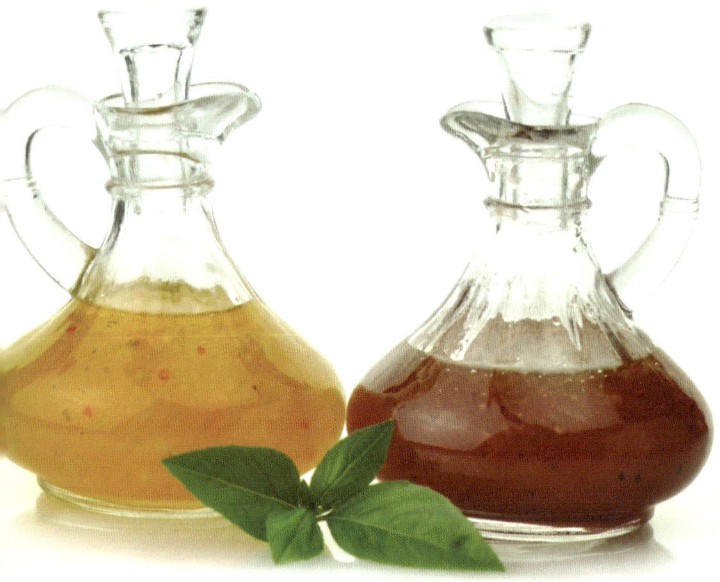

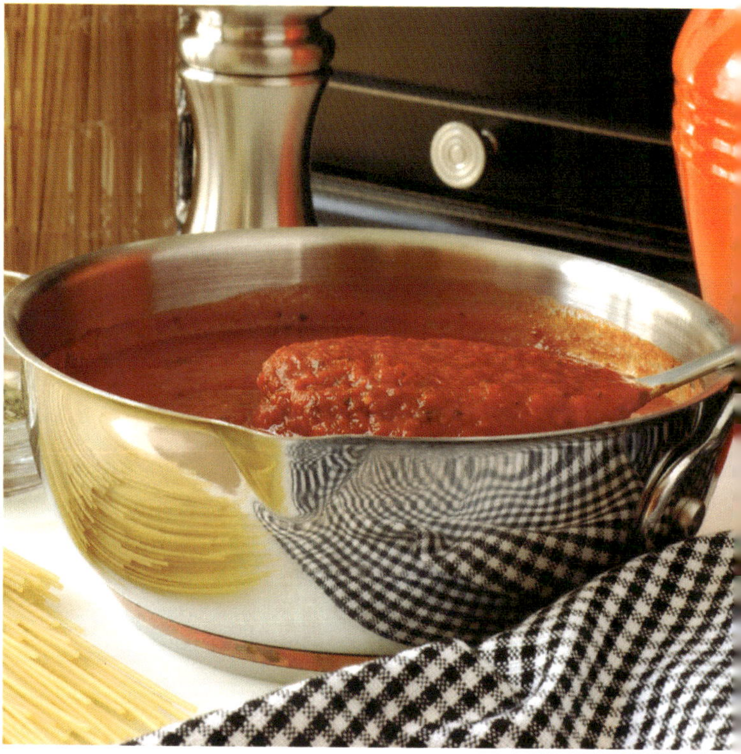

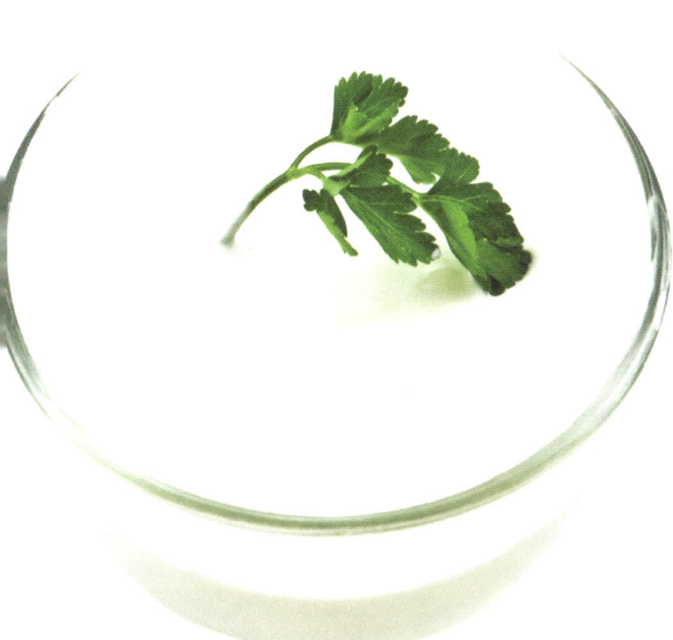 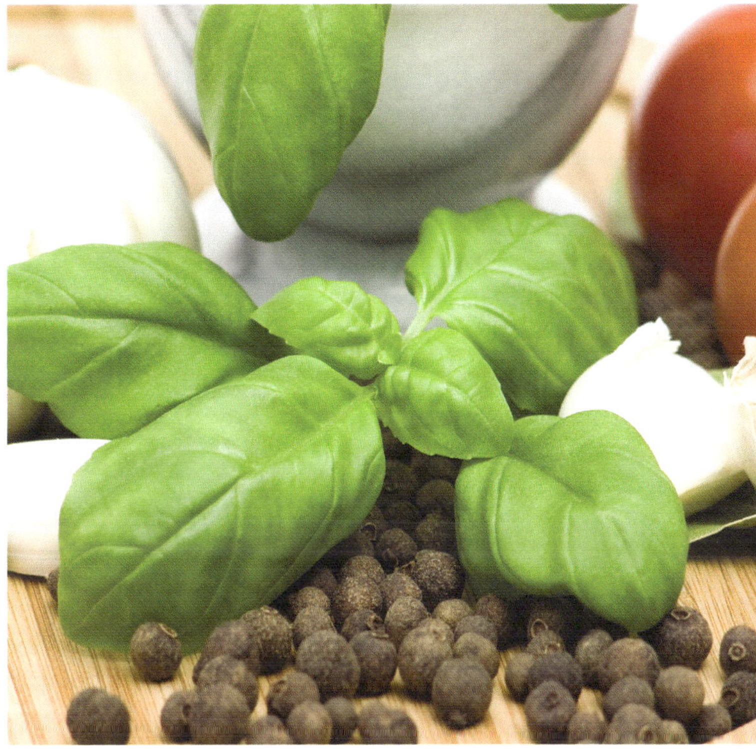

Sauces & Accompaniments

Tofu Sour Cream

1 tbs. olive oil

5 tsp. lemon juice

2 tsp. apple cider vinegar

½ tsp. salt

¼ tsp. black pepper

1 package Silken Lite Firm Tofu (10 oz.)

Instructions

In an electric blender add tofu, olive oil, lemon juice, vinegar, salt, and pepper. Place lid on blender and process until very smooth and creamy. Blend well to avoid any lumps in the mixture; it should be a smooth, sour cream-like consistency.

Tip: If you want to make French onion dip, add 1 tablespoon of dried onions and blend in the food processor until very smooth and creamy.

Serving Size: 4

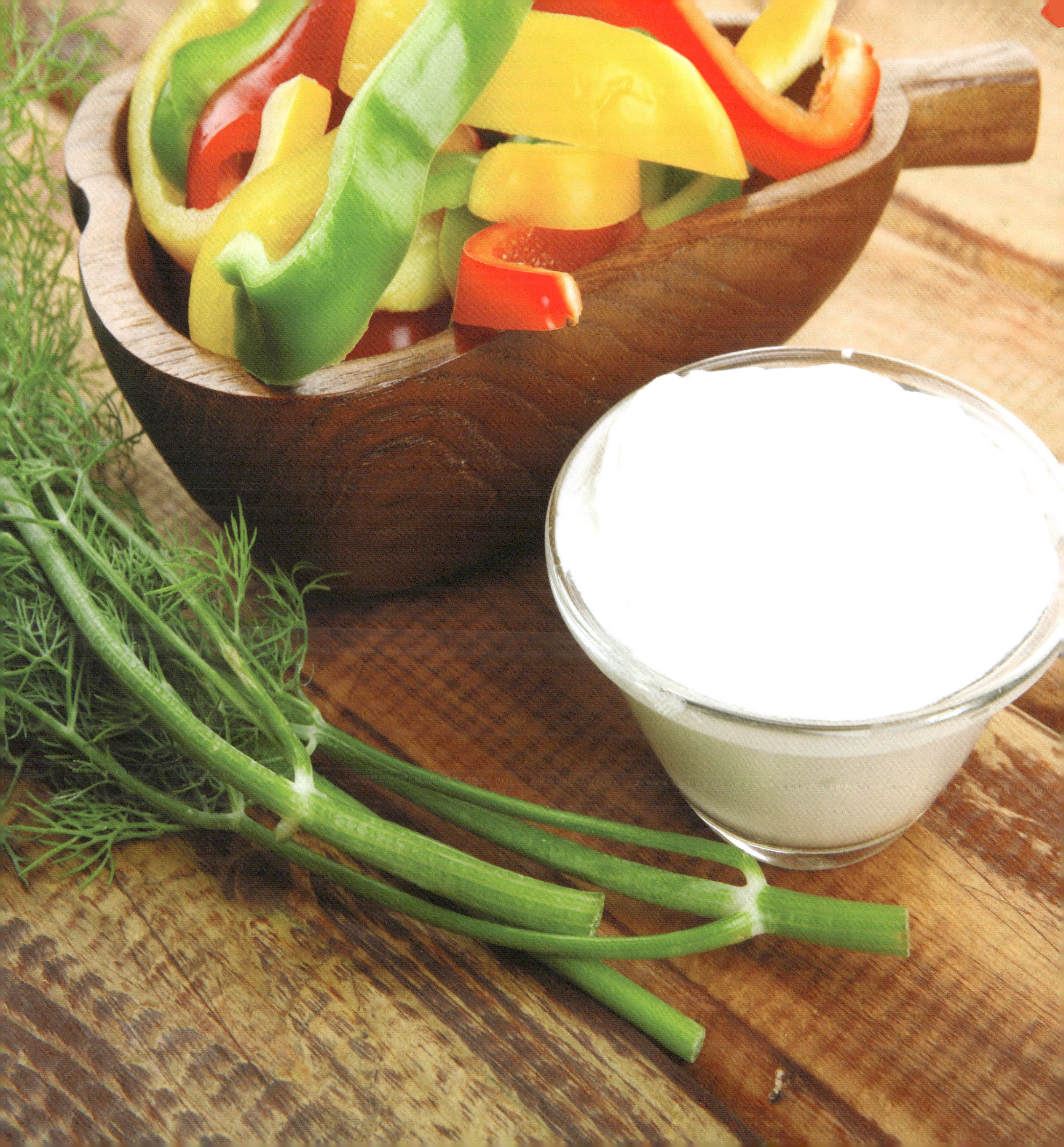

Hot Cha

3-4 green onion stalks, chopped

½ cup cold water

1 large red tomato, diced

¼ cup white or apple cider vinegar

Instructions

Prepare green onions and tomatoes as instructed. In a large bowl combine tomatoes, green onions, vinegar and water. Stir to ensure items are incorporated. Chill mixture for 1-2 hours to allow the items to incorporate.

Tip: This is a great topper for any vegetables side. Add hot cha to sautéed spinach or greens.

Serving Size: 4

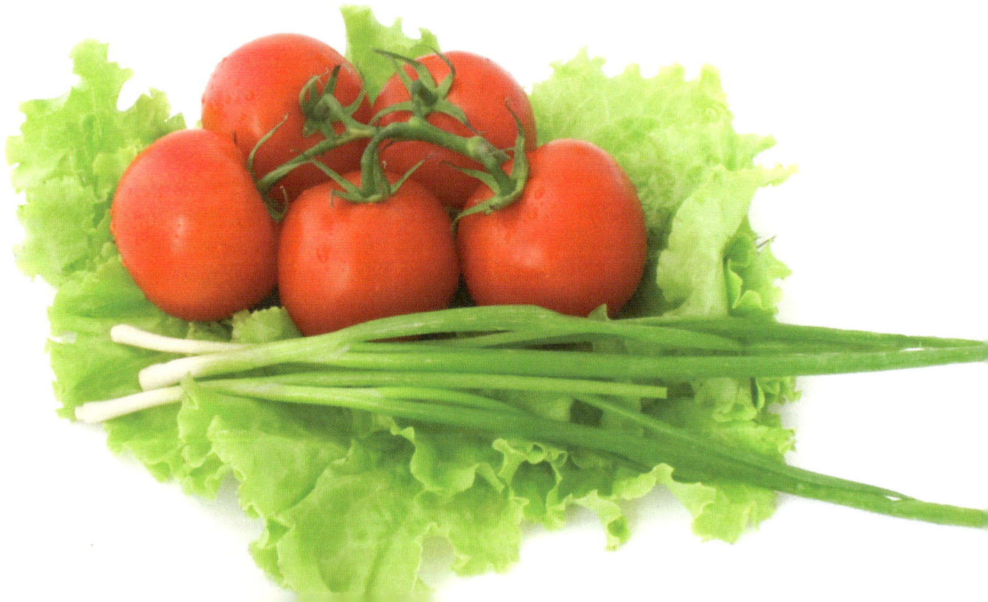

Raspberry Vinaigrette

1 pint raspberries

½ orange, juiced

2 tbs. apple cider vinegar

Kosher salt & pepper to taste

½ lemon, juiced

¼ cup water

⅓ cup olive oil

Instructions

In a small stockpot combine raspberries and water and heat over medium-high heat until raspberries release their juices. Remove from heat and strain mixture in a bowl to remove seeds. Place raspberry mixture in a blender an add vinegar, lemon, and orange juice. Blend while slowly adding olive oil. Add salt and pepper to taste.

Tip: Add additional orange or lemon juice to taste depending on how sweet or bitter the raspberries are.

Serving Size: 6

Balsamic Vinaigrette

1 shallot, minced

½ tsp. kosher salt

¾ cup olive oil

1 tbs. garlic, chopped

½ tsp. black pepper

¼ cup balsamic vinegar

Instructions

Prepare garlic and shallots as instructed. In a bowl add shallot, garlic, salt, pepper, and balsamic vinegar. Slowly pour in olive oil while whisking ingredients constantly. Taste vinaigrette to make sure you have the right balance of seasoning. Season to taste.

Tip: When you have completed the Daniel Fast, you can adjust this recipe by eliminating the garlic and adding 2 teaspoons of Dijon mustard and 2 tablespoons of honey for a delicious balsamic vinaigrette over baby spinach.

Serving Size: 4

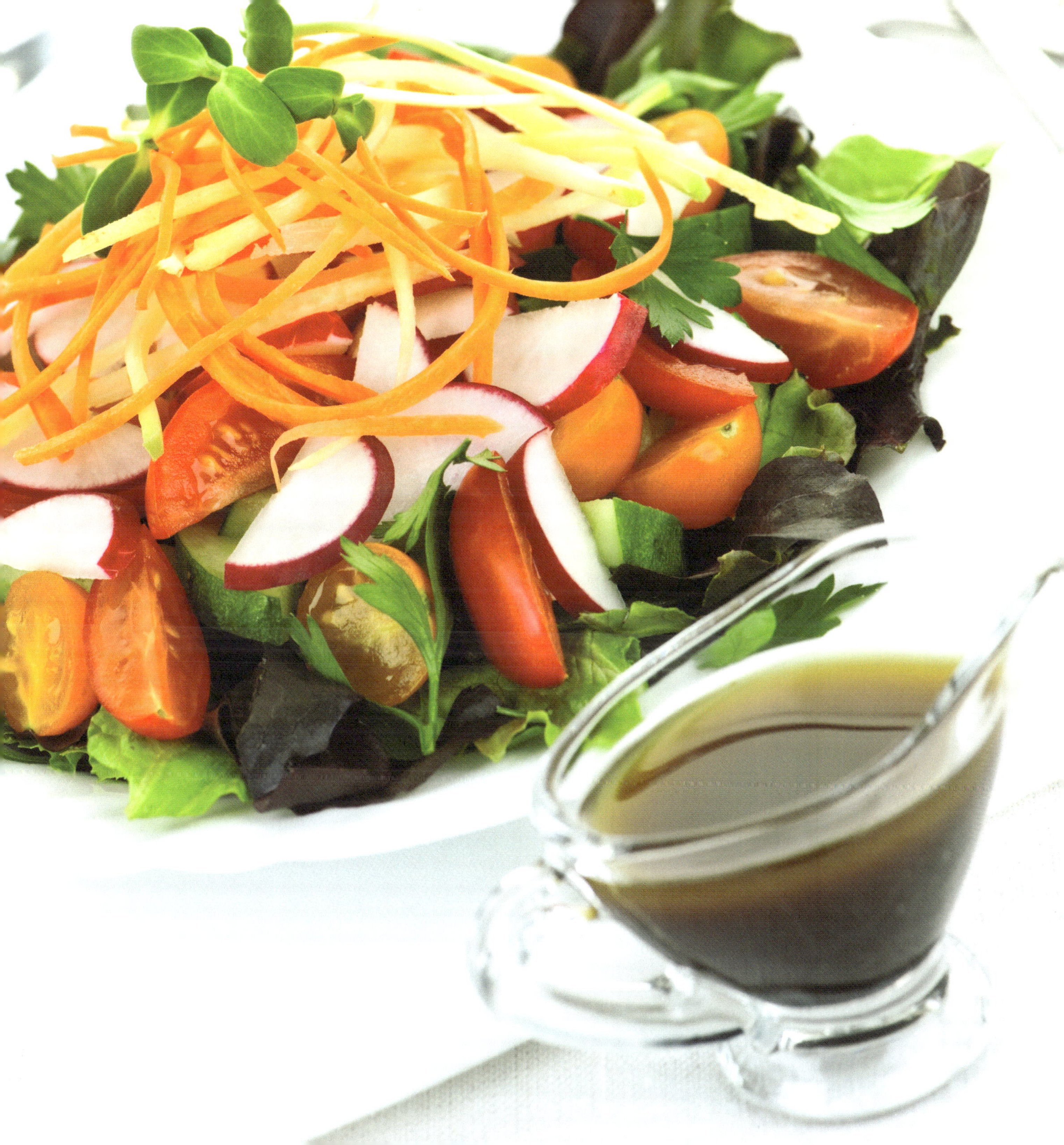

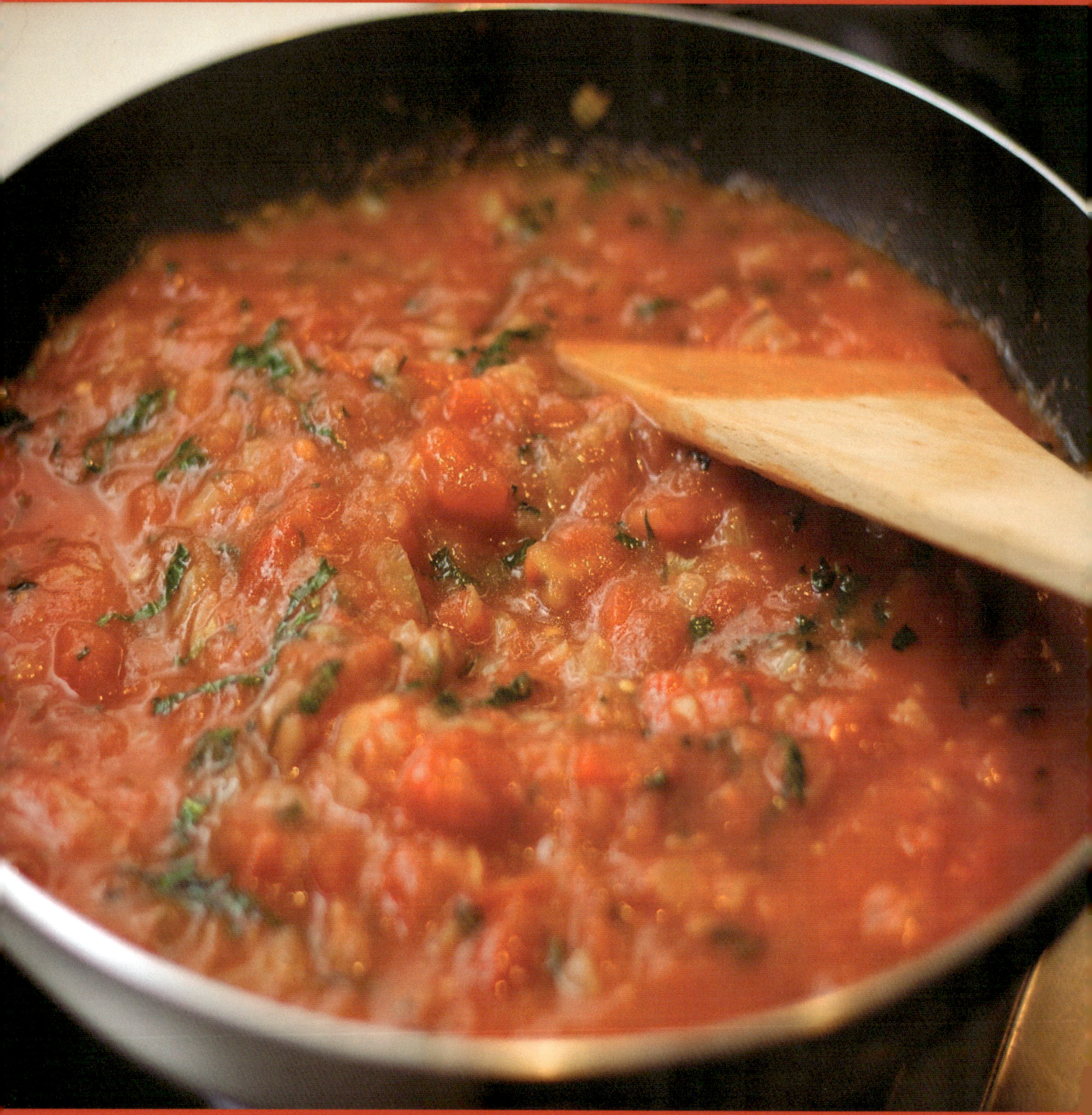

Homemade Marinara Sauce

1 large shallot, minced

4 garlic cloves, minced

1 ½ tsp. Italian seasoning

2 tbs. extra virgin olive oil

½ tsp. black pepper

1 tsp. kosher salt

1 can crushed tomatoes (San Marzano is preferred)

Instructions

Prepare shallots and garlic as instructed. In a large stockpot heat olive oil on medium-high heat and sauté shallots until translucent. Add garlic and cook 1-2 minutes. Add crushed tomatoes and lower temperature to a simmer for 10 minutes. Add Italian seasoning, salt, and pepper. If desired add more seasoning to taste.

Tip: Sauté vegetables in olive oil (e.g., mushrooms, carrots, etc.) until tender and add to sauce for a heartier marinara sauce. If you require additional sauce you can double this recipe; however, do not add additional salt or pepper.

Serving Size: 2

Roasted Red Pepper Pesto Sauce

2 red peppers, roasted and seeded

½ cup walnuts, chopped

¼ cup olive oil

½ tsp. black pepper

¾ cup fresh basil, packed

2 garlic cloves

1 tsp. kosher salt

Instructions

Preheat oven to 400 degrees. Rub red bell pepper in olive oil and roast in oven for 20-30 minutes or until skin is charred. Remove peppers from oven and place in a heat-proof bowl. Cover with plastic wrap and allow to rest for 5-10 minutes. Removed charred skin and seeds from pepper.

Add roasted peppers, basil, walnut, garlic, salt, and pepper to food processor. While blending slowly, add olive oil through feed tube.

Tip: This pesto sauce can be used as a great appetizer after the fast. Spread the roasted red pepper pesto sauce on a toasted pita chip or toss the pesto sauce in prepared whole wheat penne pasta.

Serving Size: 2

Garlic Infused Oil

1 ½ cup olive oil

6 whole garlic cloves, peeled

Instructions

Add olive oil to stockpot and heat on medium-high heat. Do not allow the oil to boil. Add peeled garlic cloves and simmer in oil for 1-2 minutes. The garlic will start to brown slightly, so make sure not to let it burn. Remove the oil from the heat and allow the garlic to infuse the olive oil until cooled completely. Remove the garlic cloves and discard. Place the garlic-infused oil in an airtight glass canning jar.

Tip: This oil is very versatile and can be used in a variety of recipes that call for olive oil and garlic.

Serving Size: 6

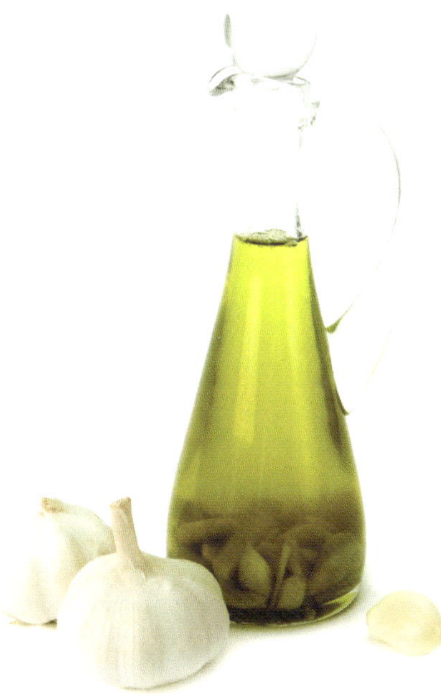

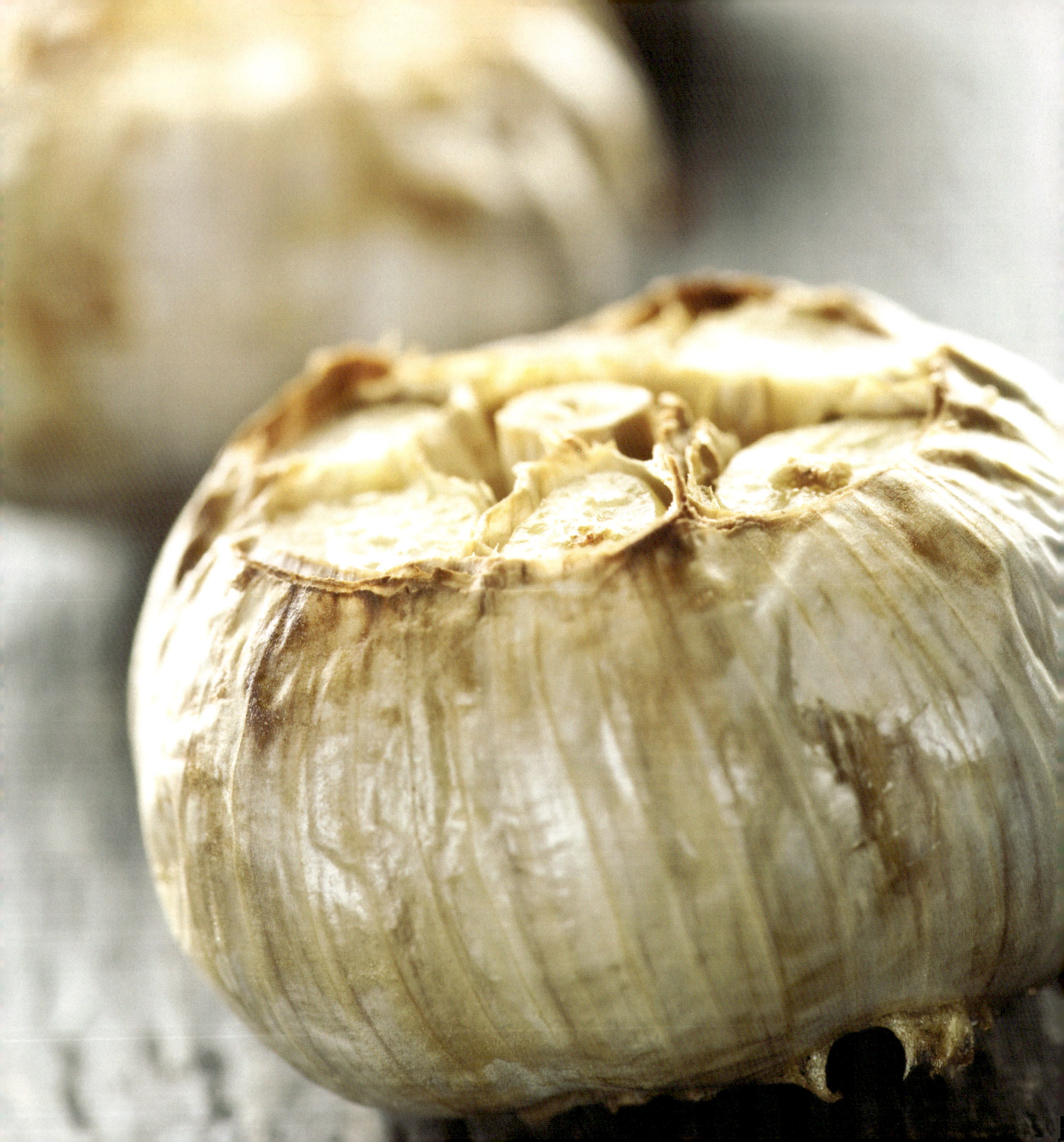

Roasted Garlic

1 garlic bulb

1 tsp. olive oil

Instructions

Preheat oven to 375 degrees. Cut top third of garlic bulb off and place in a small, round, ovenproof dish. Cover top of cut garlic bulb with olive oil. Roast in oven for 30-45 minutes until garlic is lightly browned. Remove from oven and allow the garlic bulb to cool slightly. Peel roasted garlic cloves from skin and cut or smash cloves. Add prepared cloves to your favorite dish.

Tip: Add roasted garlic to mashed potatoes to enhance flavor.

Serving Size: 1

"Even now," declares the LORD, "Return to me with all your heart, with fasting and weeping and mourning." Rend your heart and not your garments. Return to the LORD your God, for he is gracious and compassionate, slow to anger and abounding in love, and he relents from sending calamity. Joel 2:12-13 NIV

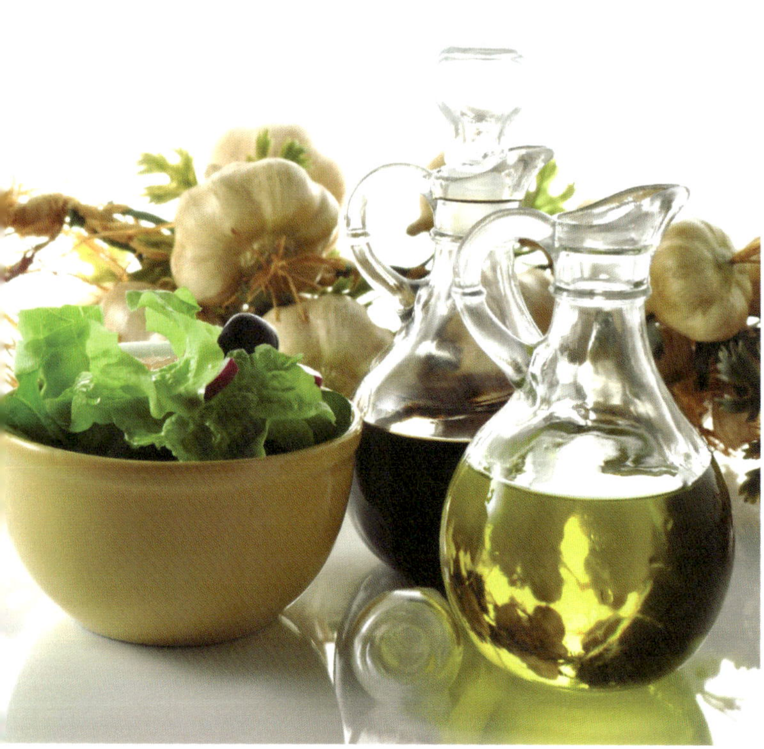

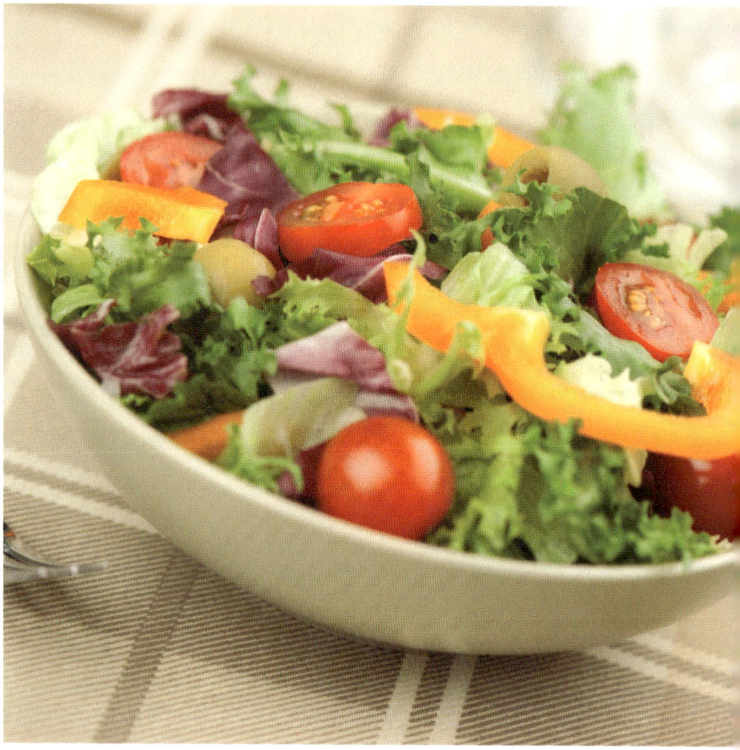

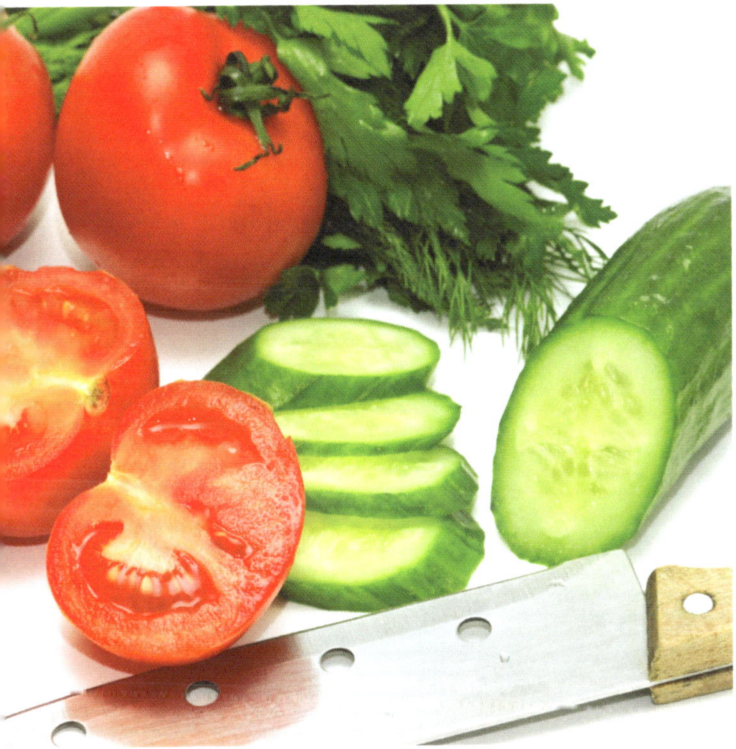

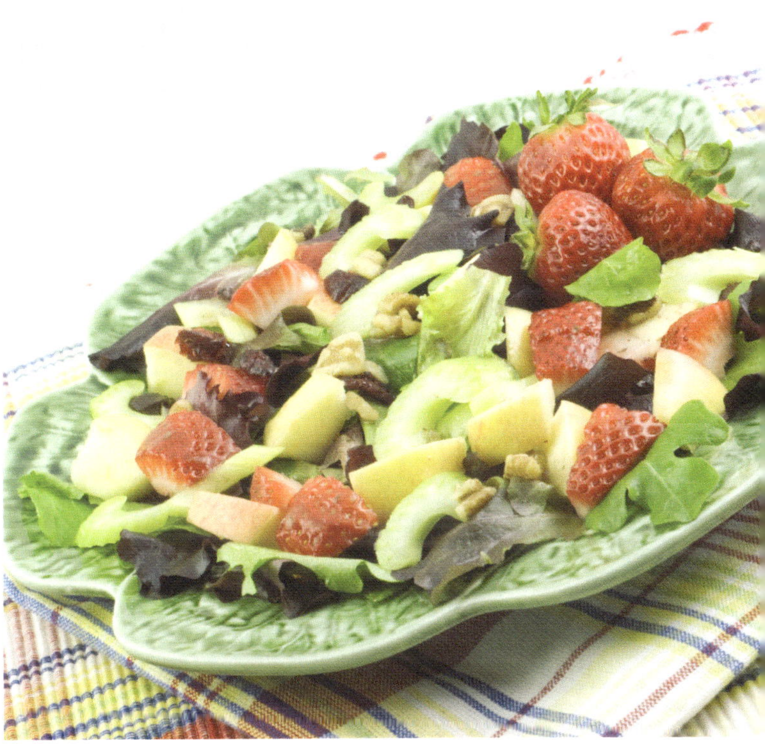

Salads

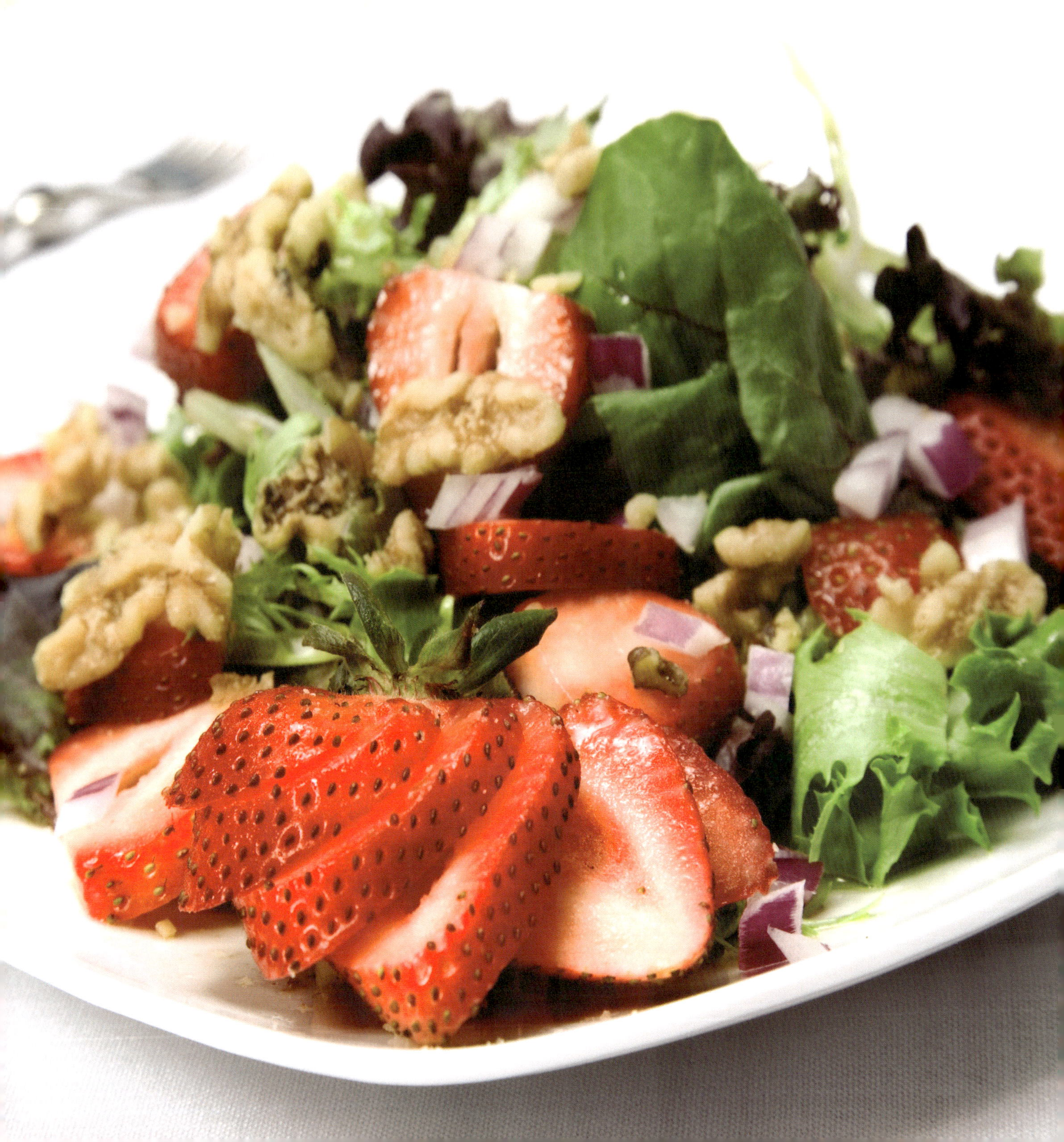

Berry Walnuts Salad

1 bag Mesclun salad mix

1 pint strawberries, sliced

Balsamic vinaigrette (see recipe on page 50)

1 cup whole walnuts

Salt & pepper to taste

Instructions

In a large ungreased frying pan, add the walnuts and heat over medium heat for 1-2 minutes to allow the essential oils to be released. Be sure to watch closely as they will burn quickly. You may want to use a wooden spoon to toss the walnuts while they are cooking. Allow the walnuts to cool completely before placing on salad greens. In a large bowl combine salad greens and cooled walnuts. Slice strawberries into quarters and add to salad. Toss salad in balsamic vinaigrette and add salt and pepper to taste.

Tip: Nuts release essential oils when roasted. When the Daniel Fast is over, add shredded Parmesan cheese to this recipe for additional crispness and freshness.

Serving Size: 2

Tossed Green Salad

1 package mixed salad greens

½ cup onion, sliced

½ cup mushrooms, sliced

1 tomato, quartered

½ cup carrots, shredded

½ cup balsamic vinaigrette

Salt & pepper to taste

1 ripe Hass avocado, seeded and with flesh removed from skin (optional)

Instructions

In a large bowl combine salad greens, tomato, onions, carrots, and mushrooms. Cut avocado in half and remove the seed, and the flesh from skin. Slice thinly. Toss all ingredients in balsamic vinaigrette. Add salt and pepper to taste.

Tip: This recipe calls for mixed salad greens; however, you may use any salad greens. I recommend preparing this salad with baby spinach or arugula.

Serving Size: 6

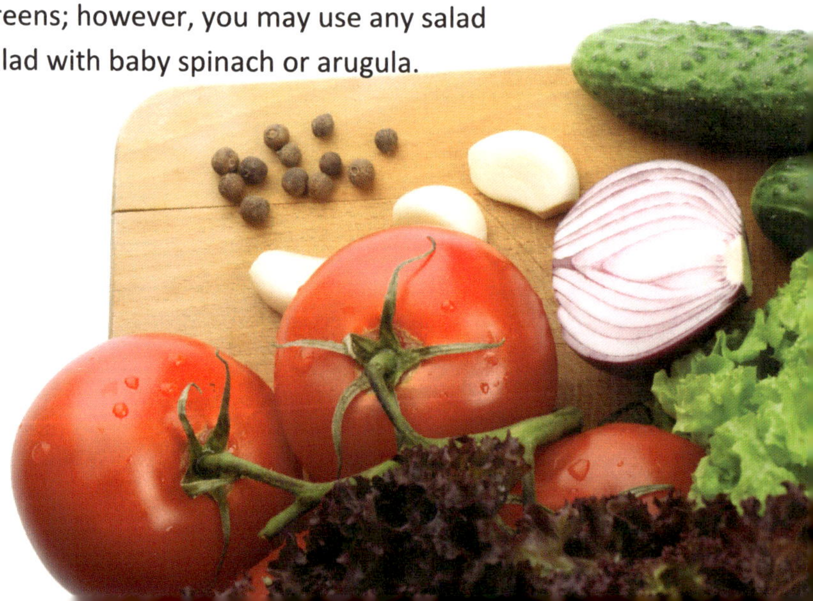

Italian Salad

1 head cauliflower

1 bunch broccoli

1 bag baby carrots

1 can green olives, drained (5.75 oz.)

1 package sliced mushrooms

1 can of medium pitted black olives, drained (6 oz.)

1 bottle Brianna's Real French Vinaigrette salad dressing

Instructions

Cut broccoli, cauliflower, and carrots into bite-sized pieces. Be sure to remove and discard the broccoli and cauliflower stems. Place the remaining florets in a large mixing bowl. Combine green olives with other ingredients. Pour salad dressing over all vegetables and mix well. Place the mixture in refrigerator overnight.

The next morning, add sliced mushrooms and black olives. Refrigerate for a couple of hours. With a large slotted spoon, drain the salad and place in another bowl. Serve salad cold or at room temperature.

Tip: This salad takes two days to make, and the longer it marinates in the dressing the better it will taste. Italian dressing is recommended for this recipe. However check the bottle to make sure it has no sugar as different brands have different ingredients.

Serving Size: 4

Romaine Salad with Pepper & Onions

1 yellow bell pepper

1 red bell pepper

2 heads of romaine lettuce

1 tsp. salt

1 orange bell pepper

1 medium sweet onion

2 tbs. olive oil

½ tsp. black pepper

Instructions

Preheat oven to 400 degrees. Remove top and seeds from bell peppers and dice into quarter inch strips. Remove onion skin and cut into large wedges, keeping the root end of the onion. On a baking sheet, combine peppers and onions. Pour olive oil over vegetables and add salt and pepper. Roast for 20-25 minutes until peppers are tender.

Slice lettuce heads in half and place on a serving platter. Remove root end of roasted onions and discard. Arrange roasted peppers and onions on top of the lettuce. Drizzle balsamic vinaigrette (see page 50 for recipe) over salad to add extra flavor.

Serving Size: 4

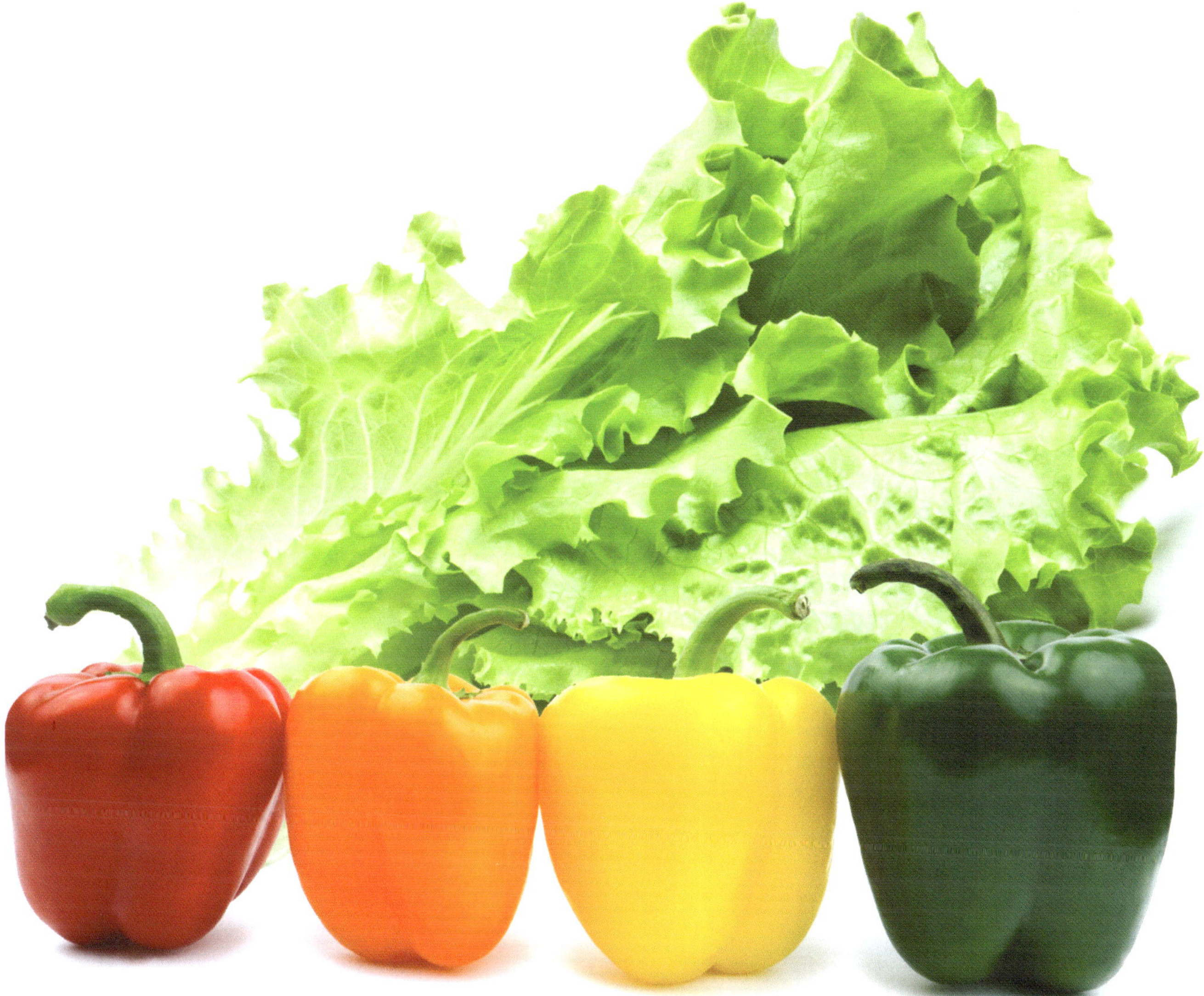

Tip: Remaining roasted vegetables can be used as a side dish to accompany any meal, or they can be used as filling for vegetable lettuce wraps.

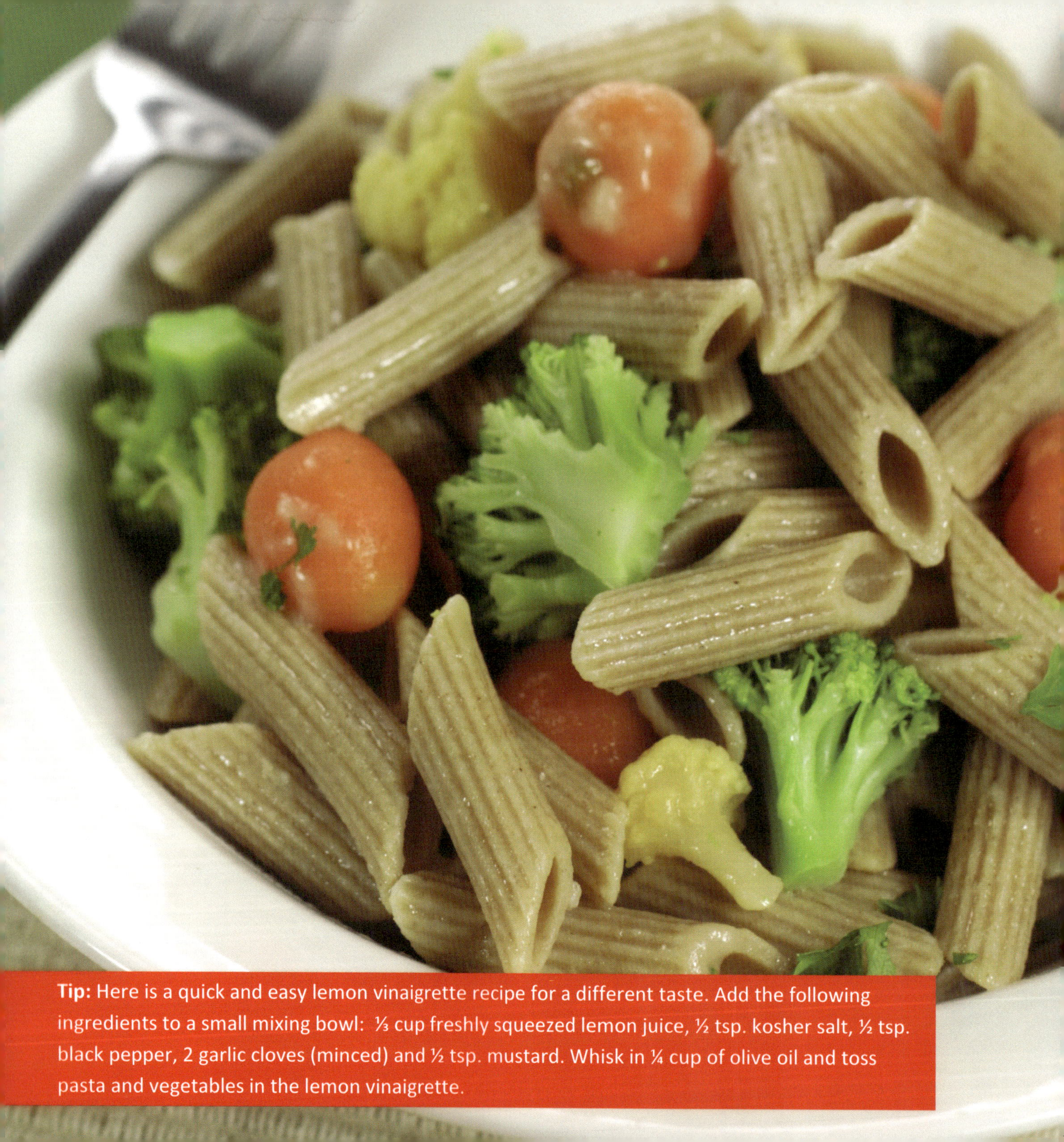

Tip: Here is a quick and easy lemon vinaigrette recipe for a different taste. Add the following ingredients to a small mixing bowl: ⅓ cup freshly squeezed lemon juice, ½ tsp. kosher salt, ½ tsp. black pepper, 2 garlic cloves (minced) and ½ tsp. mustard. Whisk in ¼ cup of olive oil and toss pasta and vegetables in the lemon vinaigrette.

Pasta Salad with Balsamic Vinaigrette

1 box Ronzoni Healthy Harvest whole grain penne rigate (13.25 oz.)

1 bag Birdseye Frozen Steam Fresh broccoli & cauliflower mix (12 oz.)

3 tbs. balsamic vinaigrette (see recipe on page 50)

1 pint cherry tomatoes, cut in half

5 quarts of water

Instructions

In a large stockpot add water and 1 tbs. kosher salt. Bring water to a boil and add penne pasta; cook for 9-10 minutes, then drain and set aside. Microwave frozen broccoli and cauliflower for 6 minutes (per package instructions). Combine cooked vegetables with penne pasta in a large mixing bowl. Slice cherry tomatoes in half and add to penne and vegetable mixture. Toss pasta salad in balsamic vinaigrette. See page 50 for recipe.

Serving Size: 4

Therefore, I urge you, brothers and sisters, in view of God's mercy, to offer your bodies as a living sacrifice, holy and pleasing to God -this is your true and proper worship. Romans 12:1

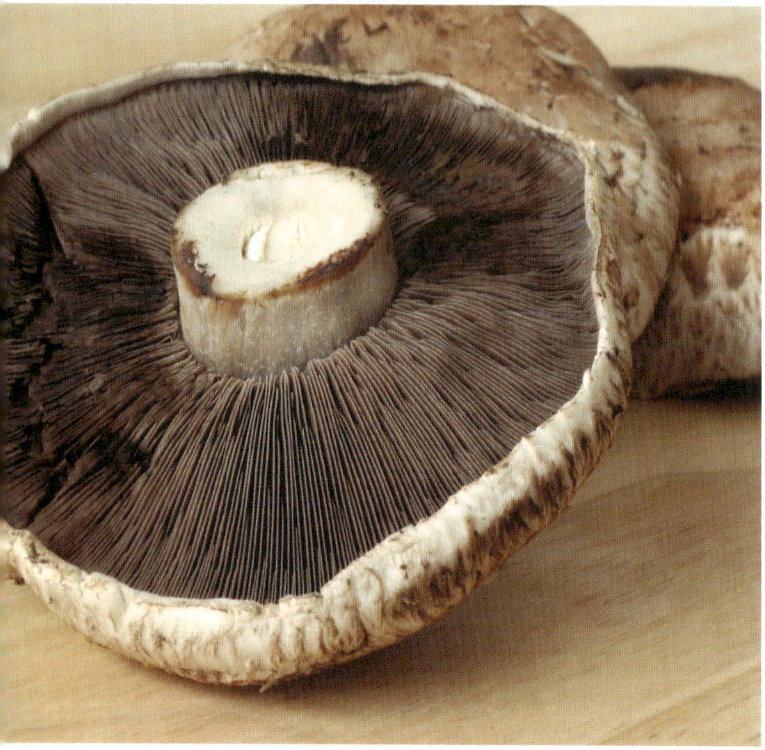

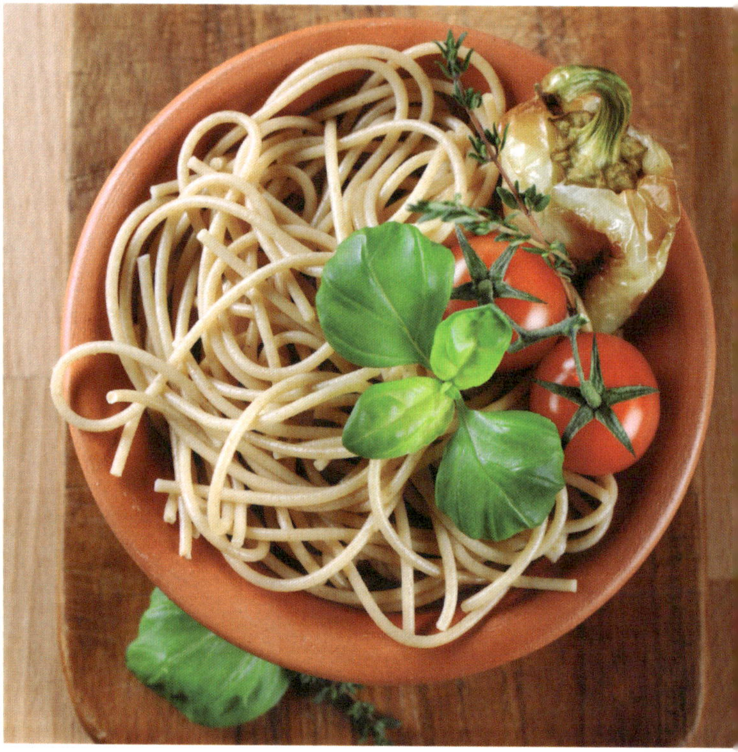

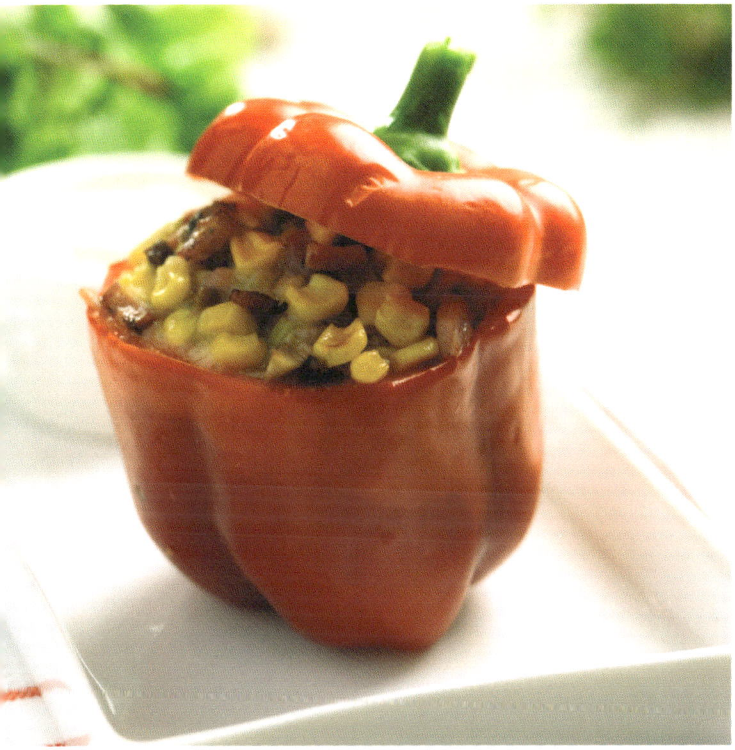

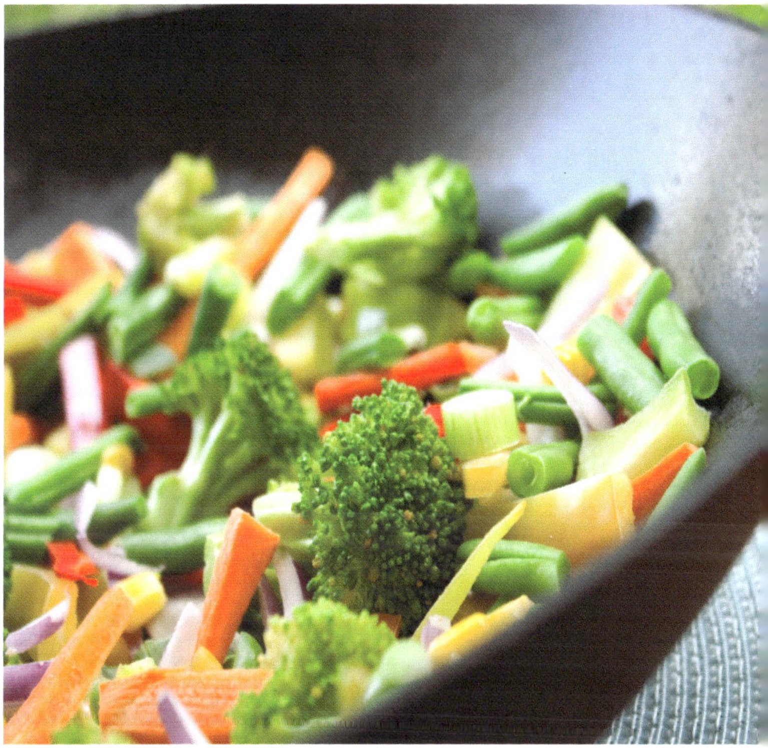

Main Dishes

Vegetable Stir Fry

3 broccoli spears, stems removed

2 tbs. soy sauce

1 tsp. garlic, minced

3 small zucchini, sliced crosswise into ¼ inch pieces

3 medium carrots, sliced crosswise into ¼ inch pieces

2 medium onions, sliced crosswise into ¼ inch pieces

2 cups uncooked Uncle Ben's instant whole grain brown rice

1 tsp. peeled ginger root, minced

2 tbs. sesame seed oil

¼ cup peanut oil

1 red bell pepper, sliced

1 can baby corn (12 oz.)

1 pint mini bella mushrooms, cut diagonally

1 green onion stalk, diced

Instructions

Prepare rice according to package directions. Cut all vegetables according to directions and set aside in a large bowl. Heat large frying pan or wok to medium-high temperature and add peanut oil. Add prepared vegetables to pan and sauté for 10 minutes or until onions are translucent and other vegetables are tender. Add garlic and ginger in the last 2 minutes of cooking. Add prepared rice to vegetables, stir and heat through. Add sesame seed oil and soy sauce. Add salt and pepper to taste. Garnish with green onions.

Serving Size: 8

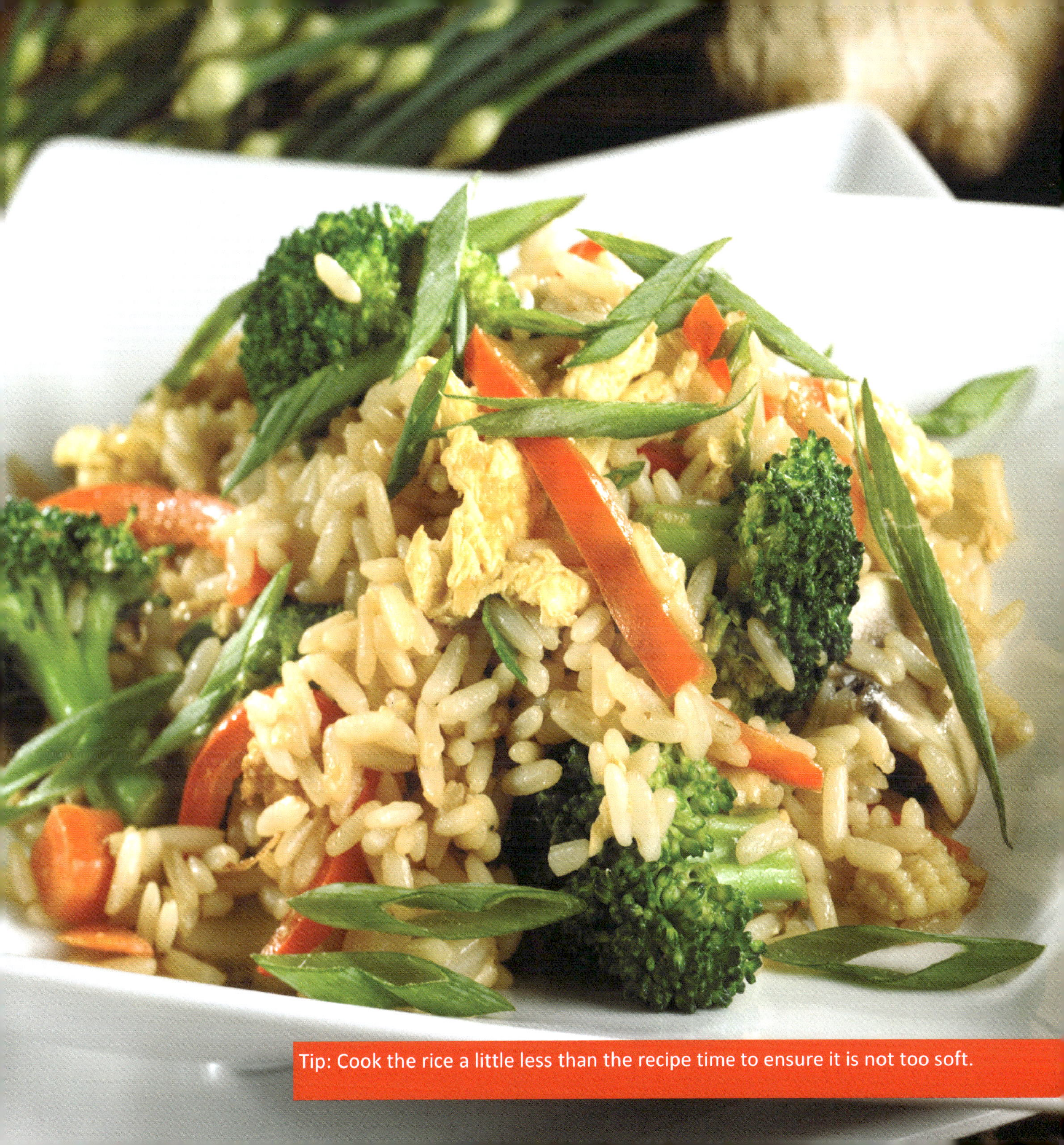

Tip: Cook the rice a little less than the recipe time to ensure it is not too soft.

Portabella Mushroom Caps with Marinara Sauce

4 large portabella mushroom caps

3 garlic cloves, minced

Vegetable cooking spray

½ tsp. kosher salt

¼ tsp. black pepper

¼ cup olive oil

2 cups homemade marinara sauce (see recipe on page 53)

Instructions

Clean mushroom caps with a damp cloth to remove dirt. Remove woody stems and discard. In a large bowl combine salt, pepper, garlic, olive oil and mushroom caps. Allow mushrooms to marinate in the mixture for 10-15 minutes. The longer the mushroom caps marinate, the more intense the flavor will be. You can prepare this recipe in either a sauté pan or griddle, but I recommend using a griddle. Heat griddle on medium-high heat on stovetop. Coat griddle thoroughly with vegetable cooking spray. Place marinated mushrooms caps on griddle and cook 6-8 minutes on each side or until mushrooms are soft and tender. You will need to flip the mushrooms caps over halfway through the cooking process to ensure even cooking. Remove mushrooms from griddle pan and place on a baking sheet. Allow mushrooms to rest for 1-2 minutes. They will release liquid during this cooling process; this is normal as mushrooms have a high moisture content. Place mushroom caps on a serving dish and ladle each with ½ cup of homemade marinara sauce.

Serving Size: 4

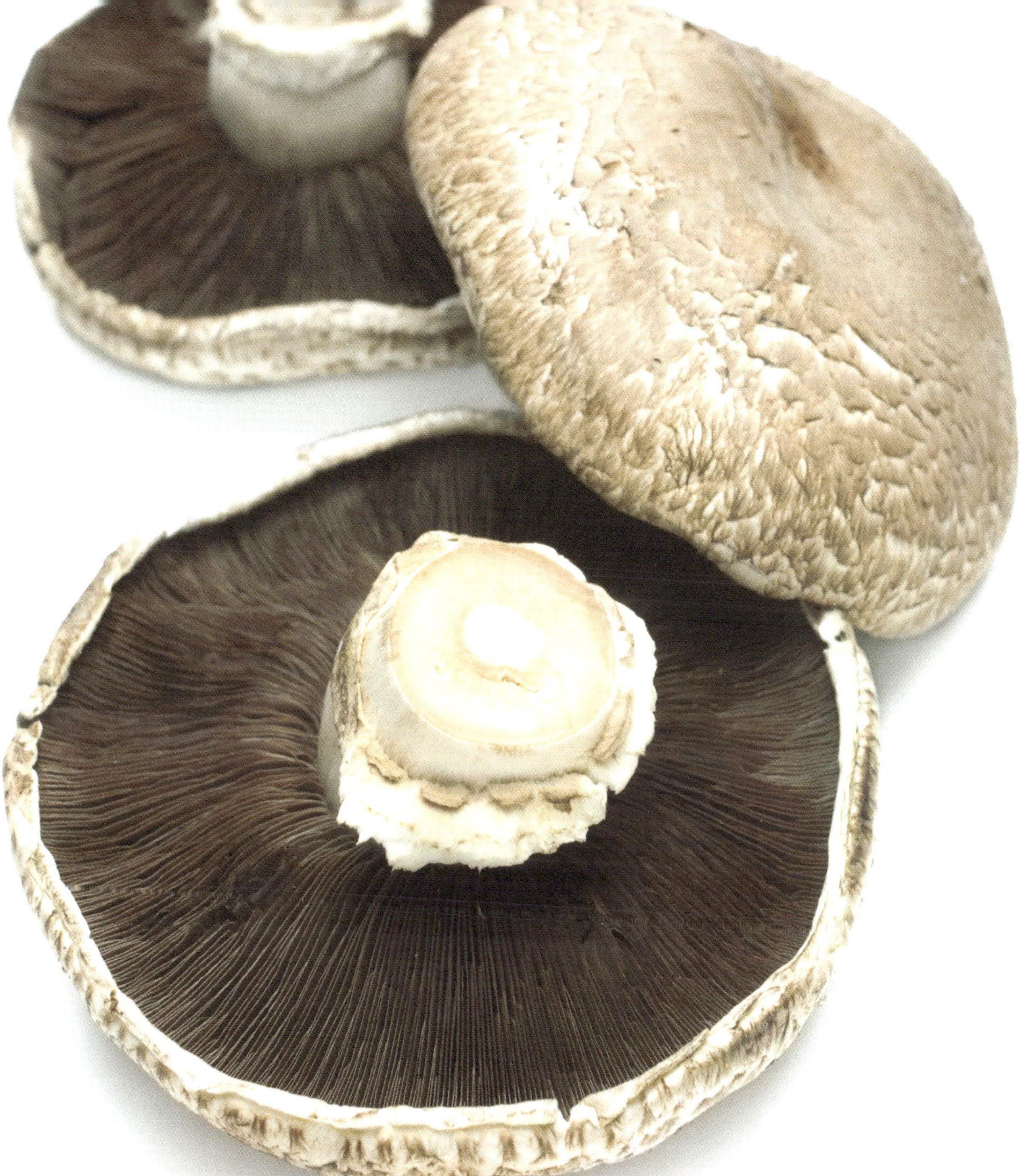

Tip: Portabella mushrooms are often referred to as vegetarian steaks due to their meaty texture. You can use prepared mushroom caps as a meat substitute in a salad.

Vegetable Stack

4 ripe tomatoes, sliced

2 large Vidalia onions, sliced

1 tbs. season salt

Vegetable cooking spray

¼ tsp. black pepper

1 bunch asparagus

½ lbs. shiitake mushrooms

¼ cup olive oil

½ tsp kosher salt

Instructions

Slice tomatoes and onions into ¼ inch rounds. Cut off woody end of asparagus spears. Place all vegetables on baking sheet and add season salt. Heat griddle on high heat and spray with vegetable spray. Cook vegetables in batches, starting with onions and ending with tomatoes, making sure that the vegetables are cooked through and are tender.

In a small skillet heat olive oil and add salt and pepper to shiitake mushrooms. Sauté mushrooms until tender. Stack vegetables on plate, starting with onion rounds, 2 spears of asparagus, and tomato rounds. Complete the stacking process two times and add the shiitake mushrooms to top of the stack.

Tip: If you don't have a griddle you can season the vegetables and roast them in a preheated oven on 400 degrees for 20-25 minutes. Follow the stacking process once vegetables are roasted.

Serving Size: 4

Vegetable Lettuce Wrap

1 yellow bell pepper

1 red bell pepper

1 medium zucchini

2 tbs. olive oil

½ tsp. black pepper

1 orange bell pepper

1 medium yellow squash

2 portabella mushroom caps

1 tsp. salt

1 head of bib lettuce leaves

Instructions

Preheat oven to 400 degrees. Remove top and seeds from all bell peppers. Cut red, yellow, and orange peppers into ¼ inch, bite-sized strips. Slice yellow squash, zucchini, and mushroom caps into medium-sized strips. Place on a baking sheet and combine bell peppers, squash, zucchini, and mushrooms; pour olive oil and add salt and pepper over vegetables. Roast in the oven for 20-25 minutes or until vegetables are tender.

Slice lettuce in half and remove core. Peel lettuce cup from head and fill with roasted vegetables. Roll lettuce around the mixture and serve.

Tip: To add extra flavor, you can prepare balsamic vinaigrette (as instructed on page 50) and use it as a dipping sauce for the vegetable lettuce wraps.

Serving Size: 4

Spaghetti Squash with Marinara Sauce

1 spaghetti squash, seeded

½ tsp. garlic powder

¼ tsp. black pepper

⅓ cup olive oil

½ tsp. kosher salt

1 cups homemade marinara sauce (see recipe on page 53)

Instructions

Preheat oven to 375 degrees. Cut spaghetti squash in half and remove the seeds. Place squash on a baking sheet cut side down. Roast spaghetti squash for 45-60 minutes or until tender. Turn squash over and use a fork to pull flesh from outer skin. The flesh will resemble long strands of spaghetti. Add the spaghetti squash to a large glass bowl and mix in olive oil, garlic powder, salt, and pepper. Toss with prepared marinara sauce.

Tip: This is a great recipe that your family will enjoy during the fast. It also is a great way to get your kids to eat vegetables because it looks so much like real spaghetti. They won't know the difference.

Serving Size: 2

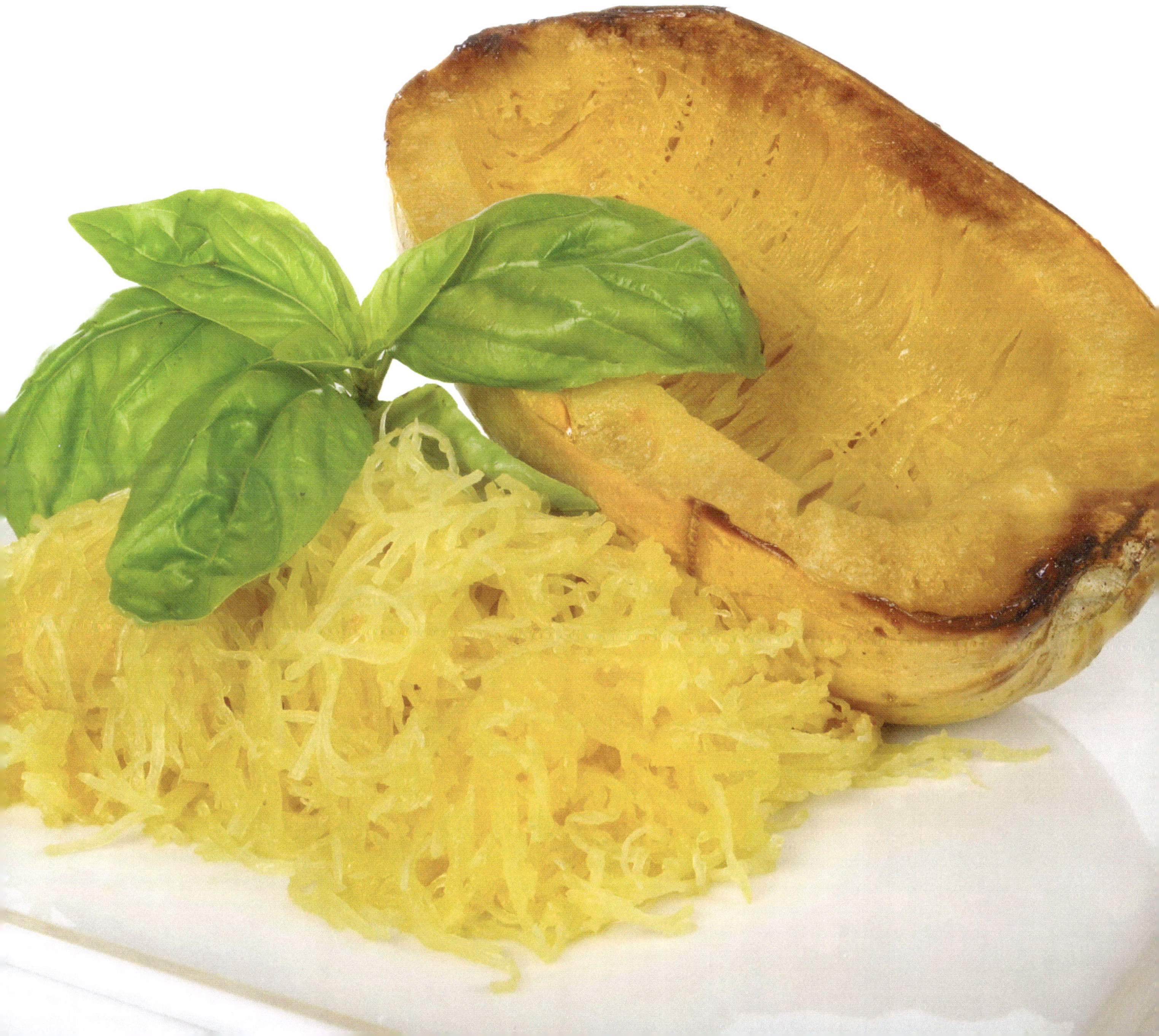

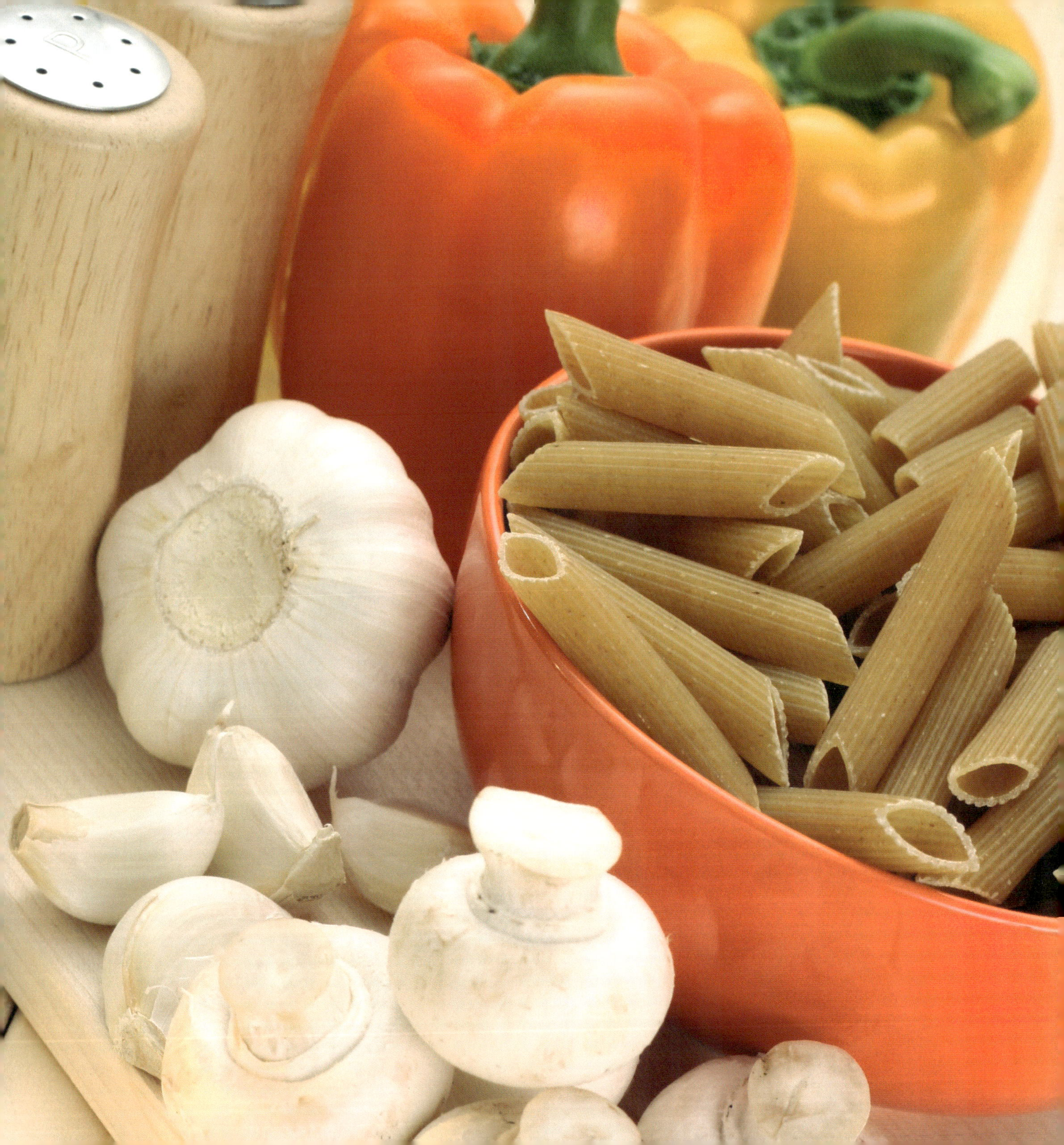

Baked Penne with Marinara Sauce

1 medium onion, diced

¼ tsp. black pepper

2 cups Veggie Shreds mozzarella cheese flavor

1 pint baby portabella mushrooms, sliced

½ tsp. kosher salt

3 garlic cloves, minced

2 tbs. olive oil

1 box whole wheat penne noodles (13.25 oz.)

2 cups homemade marinara sauce (see recipe on page 53)

Instructions

Boil pasta in large pot according to instructions for al dente. In a large skillet add olive oil. Sauté onions and mushrooms until translucent and caramelized. Add garlic in the last 1-2 minutes of cooking vegetables. Preheat oven on broil setting. In a baking dish add pasta, onions, mushrooms, and garlic. Add 2 cups of prepared marinara sauce and mix thoroughly. Top dish with mozzarella flavored cheese and allow cheese to melt under broiler for 3-5 minutes.

Tip: Different brands of whole wheat pasta will taste different. Be sure to try out several types to find the brand you like the best. Always be sure to add ½ teaspoon of kosher salt to boiling water when cooking pasta; this will make the pasta taste better.

Serving Size: 6

Eggplant Parmesan

2 large eggplants, sliced

¼ cup dried parsley flakes

½ tsp. black pepper

1 cup Veggie Shreds, mozzarella cheese flavor

1 cup corn flour

1 tsp. kosher salt

1 lb. whole wheat spaghetti (optional)

¼ cup olive oil, plus extra for sauté process

2 cups homemade marinara sauce (See recipe on page 53)

Instructions

Preheat oven to 375 degrees. Slice eggplant into ½ inch rounds. Place each round on a baking sheet and season with salt and pepper on both sides. The salt will begin to bring the moisture out of the eggplant; this moisture will allow the corn flour to stick to the eggplant. In another bowl combine corn flour and dried parsley flakes. Dredge each eggplant round in corn flour and parsley mixture. In a large sauté pan heat olive oil on medium-high. Lightly sauté floured eggplant rounds in olive oil, ensuring both side are lightly browned. You will have to repeat the sauté process multiple times for the remaining breaded eggplant. Be sure to add additional olive oil to allow the breaded eggplant to brown evenly.

Ladle prepared homemade marina sauce on the bottom of an 11" X 15" ovenproof glass baking dish. Place sautéed eggplant in two rows so that they overlap. Add a line of marinara sauce down the center of the eggplant and sprinkle mozzarella cheese on top. Place dish in oven and bake 15-20 minutes to allow the cheese to melt. If you prefer to serve the eggplant with pasta, prepare whole wheat spaghetti in boiling salted water and cook until al dente.

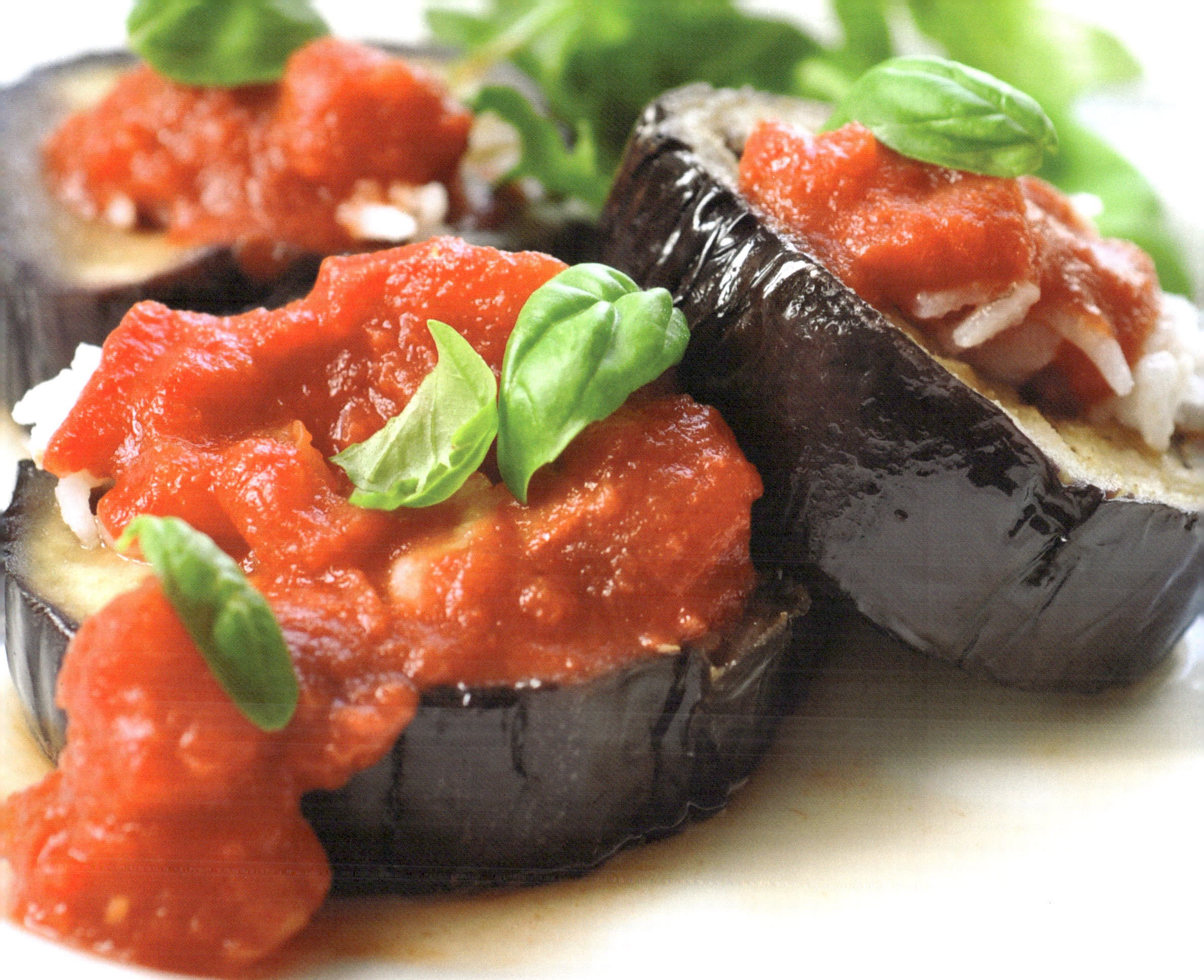

Drain spaghetti and toss in prepared homemade marinara sauce. Place spaghetti on a plate and add 1-2 slices of prepared eggplant on top. Add additional marinara sauce as desired.

Serving Size: 8

Tip: When placed in liquid, eggplant will absorb the moisture. As you sauté the eggplant you will have excess corn flour in the bottom of the pan. You may have to clean the pan out multiple times and add additional olive oil to correctly sauté the eggplant.

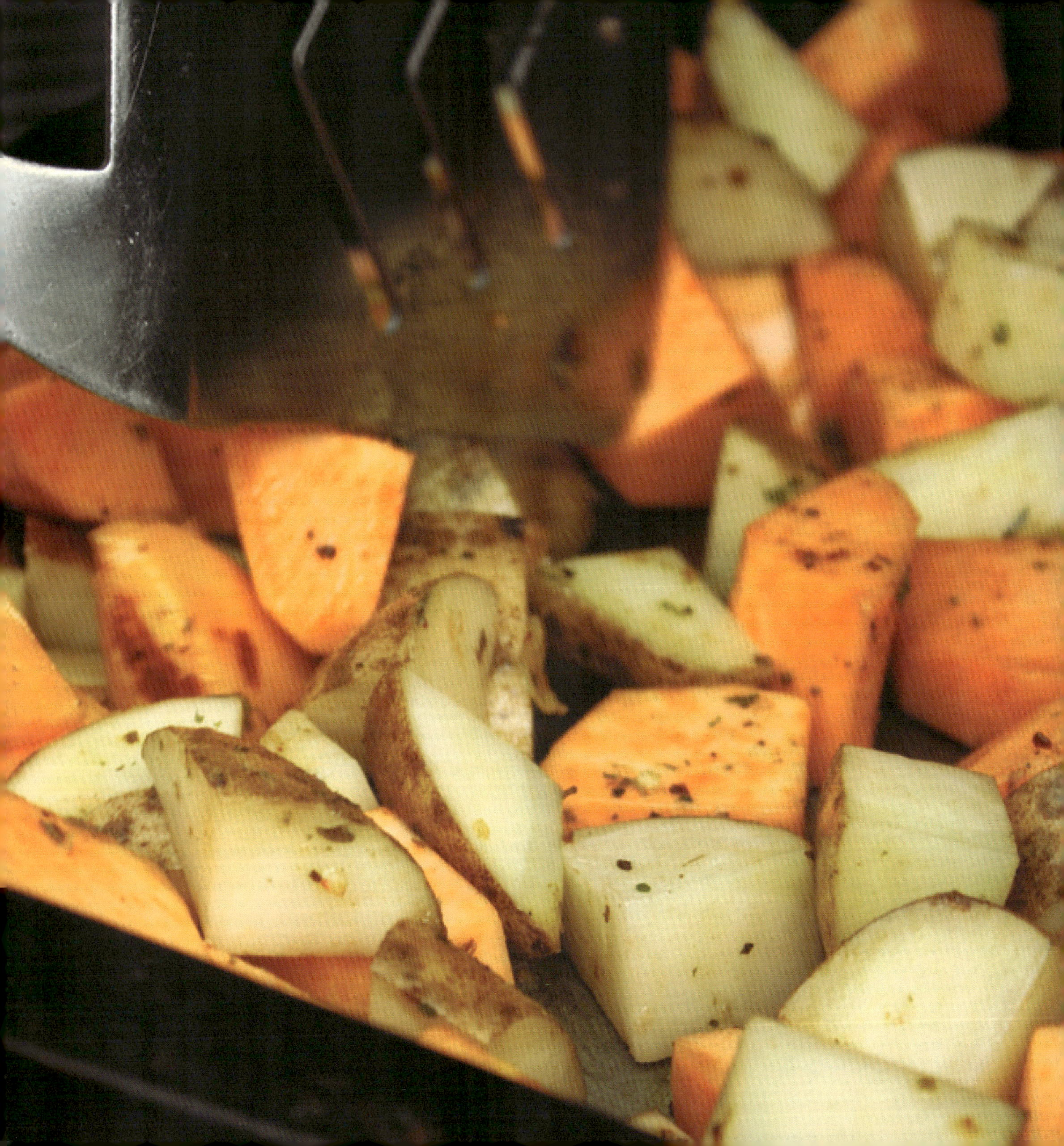

Sweet Potato Hash

1 medium onion, diced

1 yellow bell pepper, diced

½ tsp. kosher salt

4 medium sweet potatoes, peeled and cubed

1 pint sliced mushrooms

3 tbs. olive oil

¼ tsp. black pepper

2 green onion stalks, diced

Instructions

Preheat oven to 400 degrees. Prepare sweet potatoes as instructed and place on an ungreased baking sheet. Season with salt and pepper and add 1 tablespoon of olive oil to potatoes. Mix potatoes by hand, coating evenly to ensure all cut surfaces are coated with oil. Place in preheated oven for 20-30 minutes or until potatoes are tender. To test tenderness, pierce the center of potatoes with a sharp knife. If it goes through easily, they are done.

In a large frying pan add 2 tablespoons of olive oil, diced onions, mushrooms, and yellow bell pepper. Heat on medium-high heat until onions are translucent and slightly caramelized. Remove sweet potatoes from baking sheet and add to mixture in frying pan. Add additional salt and pepper to taste. Finish by adding diced green onions.

Tip: Once you are done with your fast, add cubed turkey for a heartier meal. You can also add a poached or over hard egg on top of the hash once you have completed your Daniel Fast.

Serving Size: 4

Spaghetti with Marinara Sauce

1 lb. whole wheat spaghetti

6 cups water

2 tbs. olive oil

½ tsp. salt

1 cup homemade marinara sauce (see recipe on page 53)

Instructions

Prepare homemade marinara sauce as instructed on page 53 prior to preparing spaghetti. In a large stockpot bring water, salt, and olive oil to a boil. Add whole wheat pasta and cook according to package instructions or until al dente. Drain and place ½ cup cooked pasta on a dinner plate. Add 1 cup homemade marinara sauce to cooked pasta.

Tip: Save ½ cup of pasta water when draining pasta. You may need to use this water to loosen the pasta after cooking, as it will start to stick when it becomes dry.

Serving Size: 4

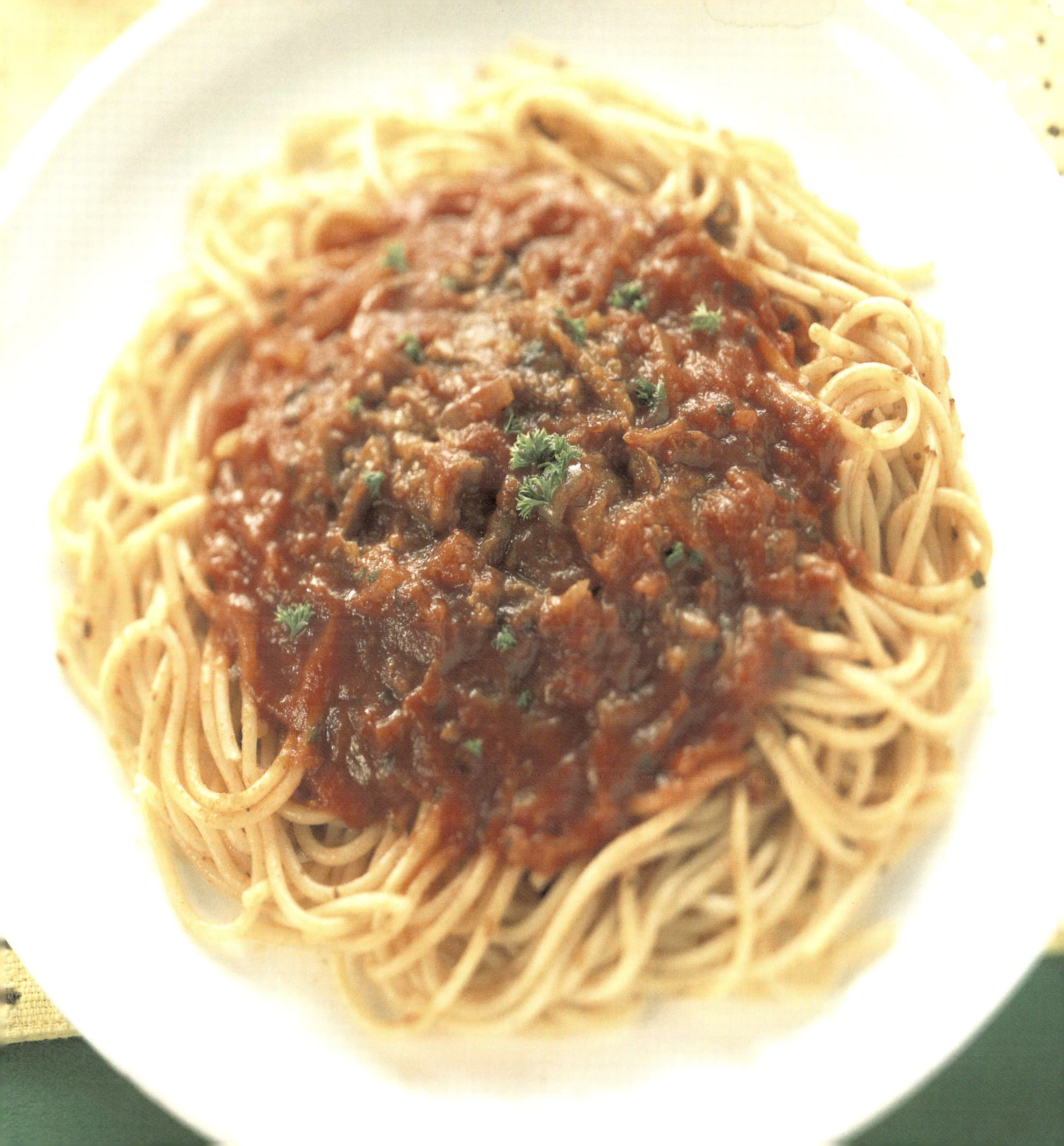

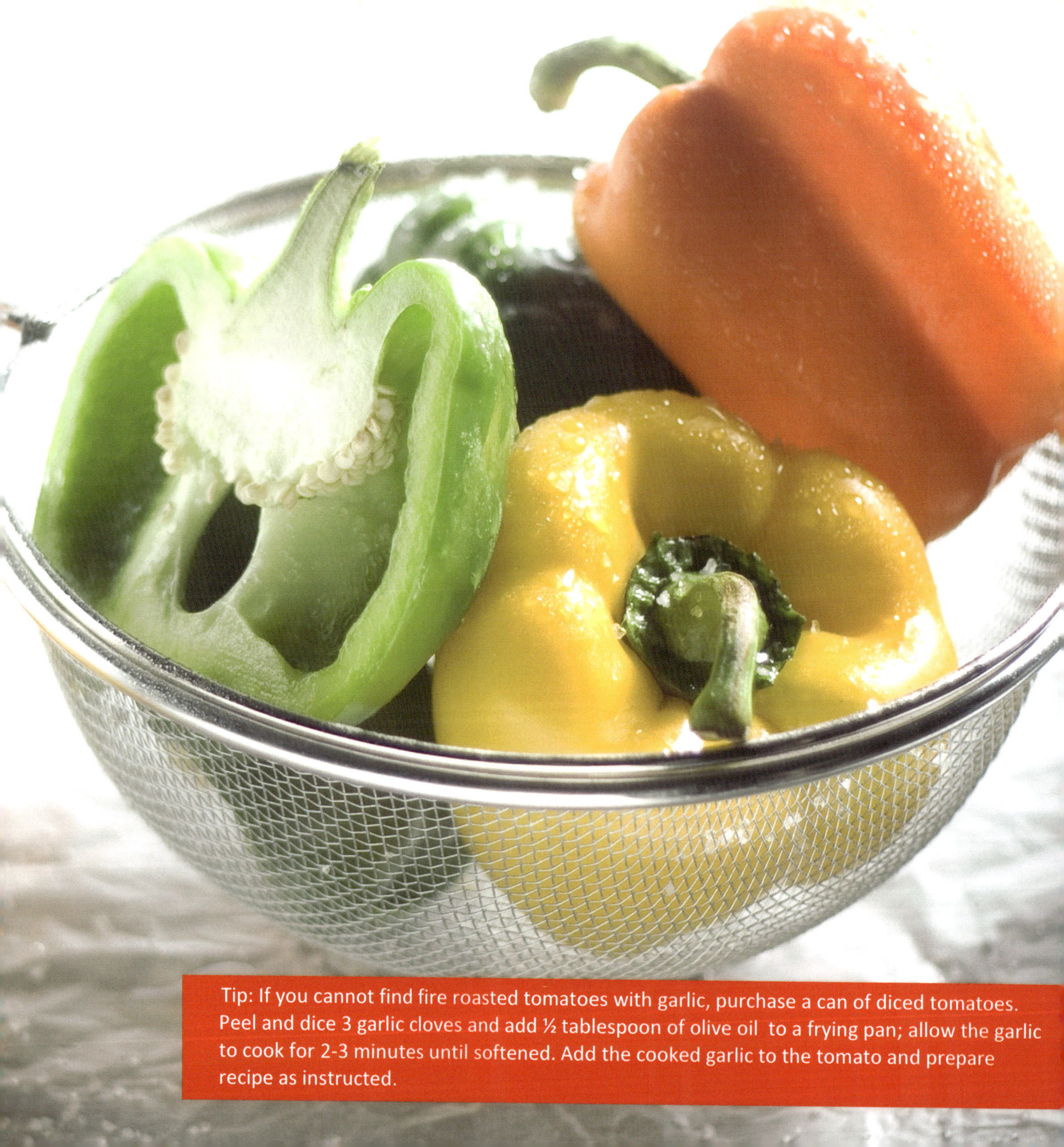

Tip: If you cannot find fire roasted tomatoes with garlic, purchase a can of diced tomatoes. Peel and dice 3 garlic cloves and add ½ tablespoon of olive oil to a frying pan; allow the garlic to cook for 2-3 minutes until softened. Add the cooked garlic to the tomato and prepare recipe as instructed.

Stuffed Peppers

9 assorted bell peppers (red, yellow, orange)

1 can Goya black beans, drained (15.5 oz.)

¼ tsp. black pepper

1 can Heinz fire roasted tomatoes with garlic (15.5 oz.)

1 cup baby spinach

½ tsp. season salt

2 cups prepared whole grain rice

Instructions

Preheat oven to 375 degrees. Cut tops off 6 bell peppers and remove seeds. Place on a baking sheet and place in oven for 10 minutes to allow the peppers to roast and soften. Remove from oven and wrap each pepper in aluminum foil. In a small stockpot prepare brown rice according to instructions on box and set aside. Drain black beans and set aside.

Chop the remaining 3 bell peppers (red, yellow, and orange) into medium-sized pieces. Add olive oil to a frying pan and add the diced onions and bell peppers to the pan. Heat over medium heat until onions are translucent and bell peppers are soft. Add season salt, black pepper, spinach, and black beans. Allow the spinach to wilt and heat the black beans completely. Add the prepared brown rice and half of the tomatoes. Unwrap the bell peppers and stuff the rice mixture into the bell peppers. Place stuffed bell pepper in glass baking dish with bell peppers upright in dish. Add the remaining fire roasted tomatoes to the top of each bell pepper. Place stuffed peppers in oven for 20 minutes, allowing all the mixture to incorporate and the bell peppers to continue to soften.

Serving Size: 6

"For I know the plans I have for you," says the LORD. "They are plans for good and not for disaster, to give you a future and a hope. In those days when you pray, I will listen. If you look for me wholeheartedly, you will find me." Jeremiah 29:11-13 NLT

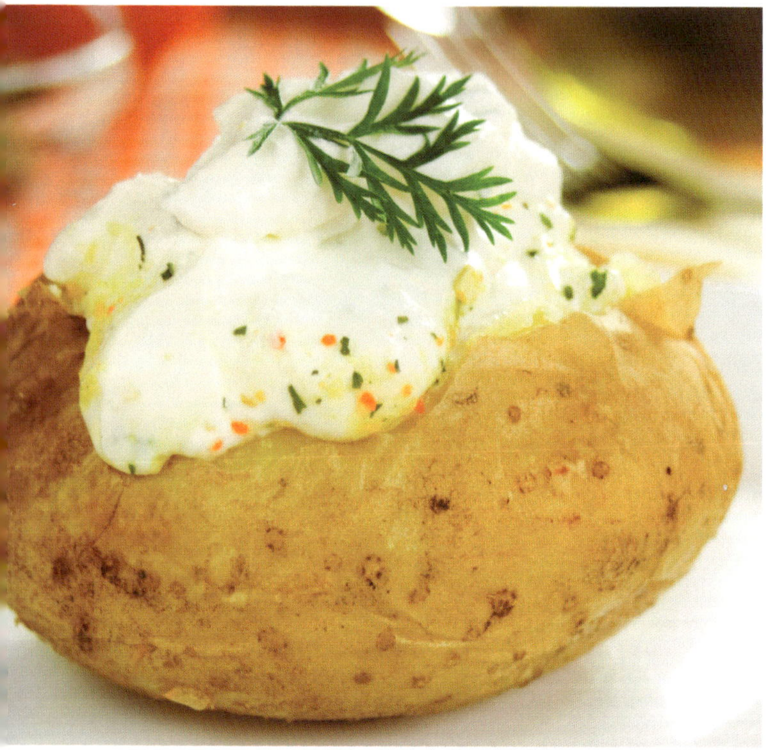

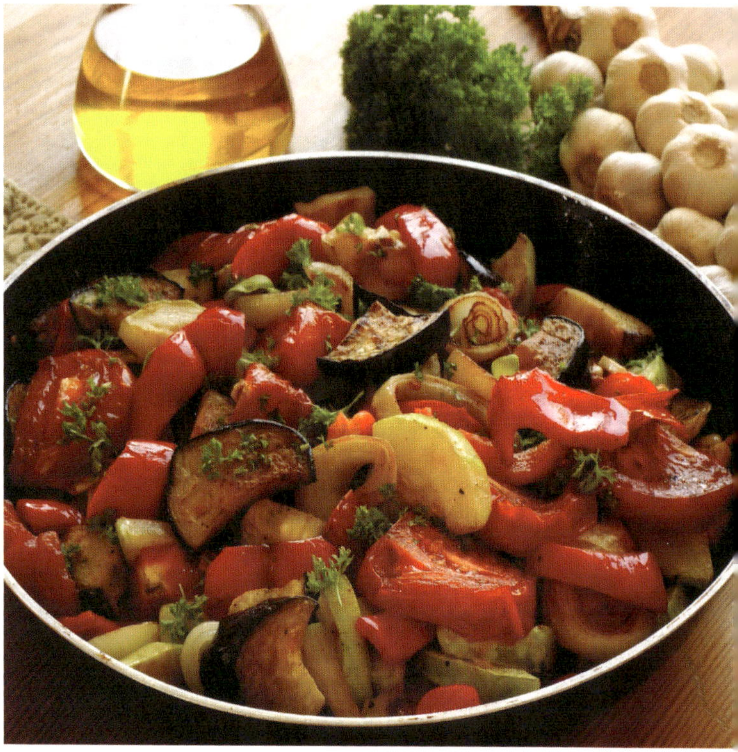

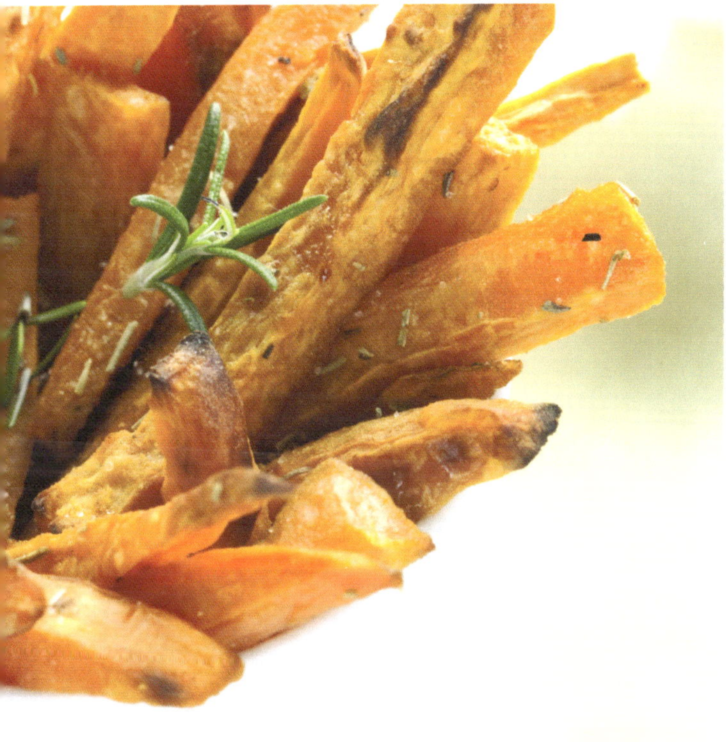

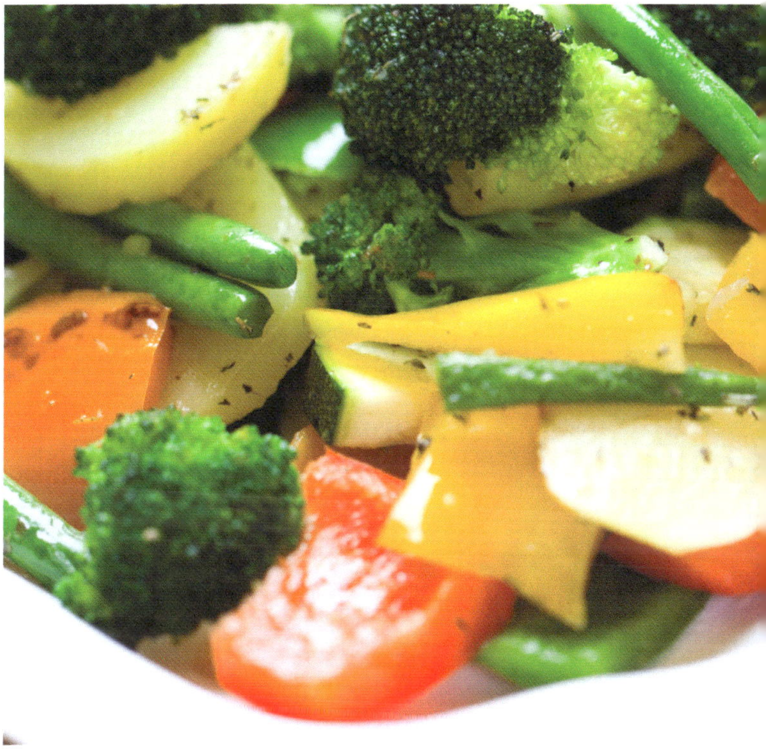

Side Dishes

Roasted Vegetables

2 large sweet onions

1 large red bell pepper

1 large yellow bell pepper

½ tbs. kosher salt

⅓ cup olive oil

1 pint whole baby bella mushrooms

1 large orange bell pepper

6 whole garlic cloves, peeled

¼ tbs. black pepper

¼ tsp. thyme

Instructions

Preheat oven to 400 degrees. If you have a convection roast setting on your oven, you can use this setting also. Cut vegetables into even sizes to ensure even roasting. Below are directions on how to cut the vegetables to achieve the desired roasting. Peel onions and cut into wedges, leaving the root end on. Next, cut tops and bottoms off the bell peppers. Remove seeds and slice lengthwise into quarter wedges. After cutting, place onions, bell peppers, mushrooms, and garlic cloves on a large baking sheet. Add salt, pepper, olive oil, and thyme. Flip vegetables halfway through cooking process to ensure all items are evenly coated. Place in oven and roast for 40-55 minutes or until vegetables are tender and the edges are brown.

Tip: This recipe requires an extensive amount of cutting to ensure that all of the items are cut to similar sizes so they roast evenly. You can replace any vegetable in this recipe with others you prefer.

Serving Size: 4

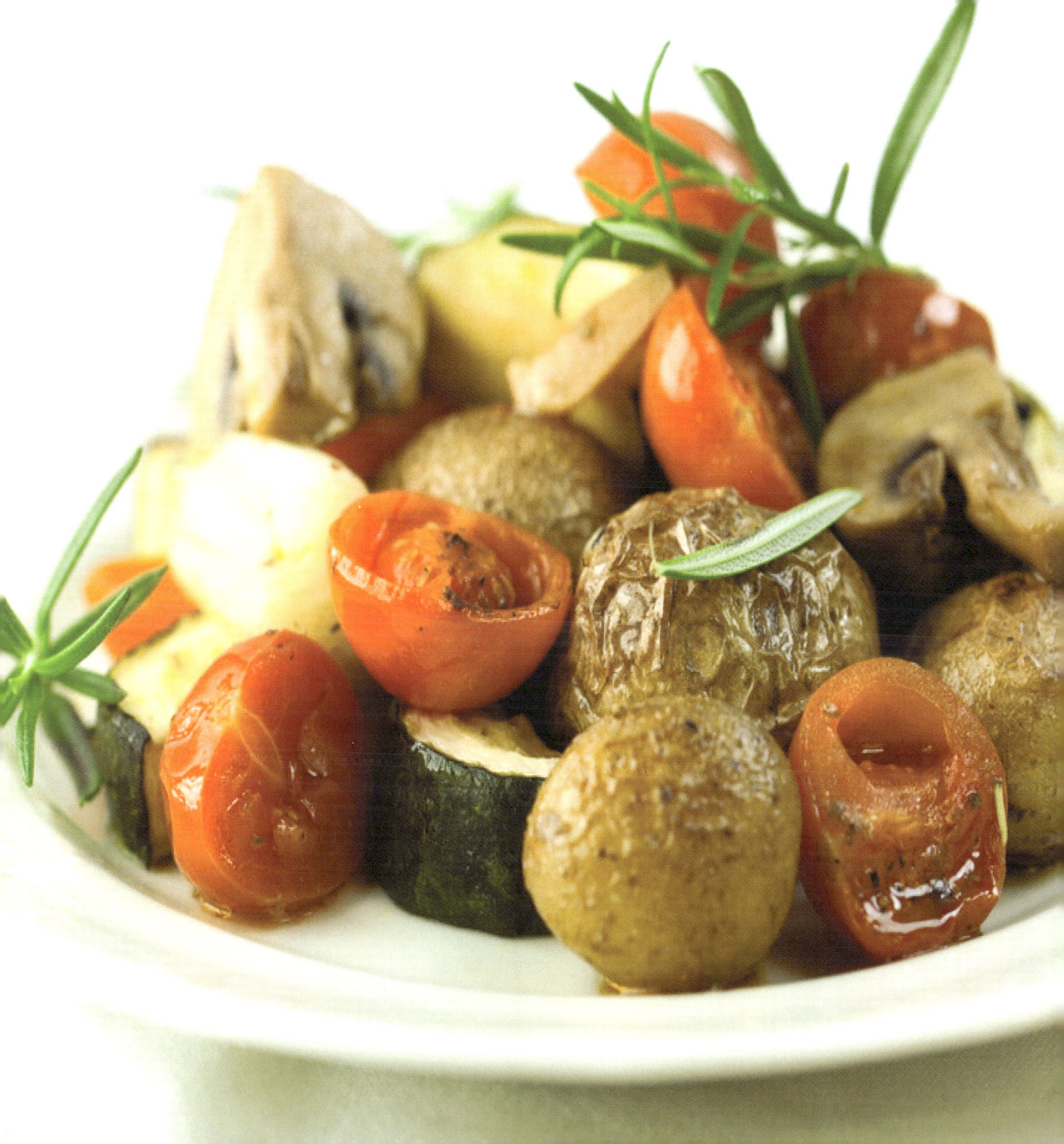

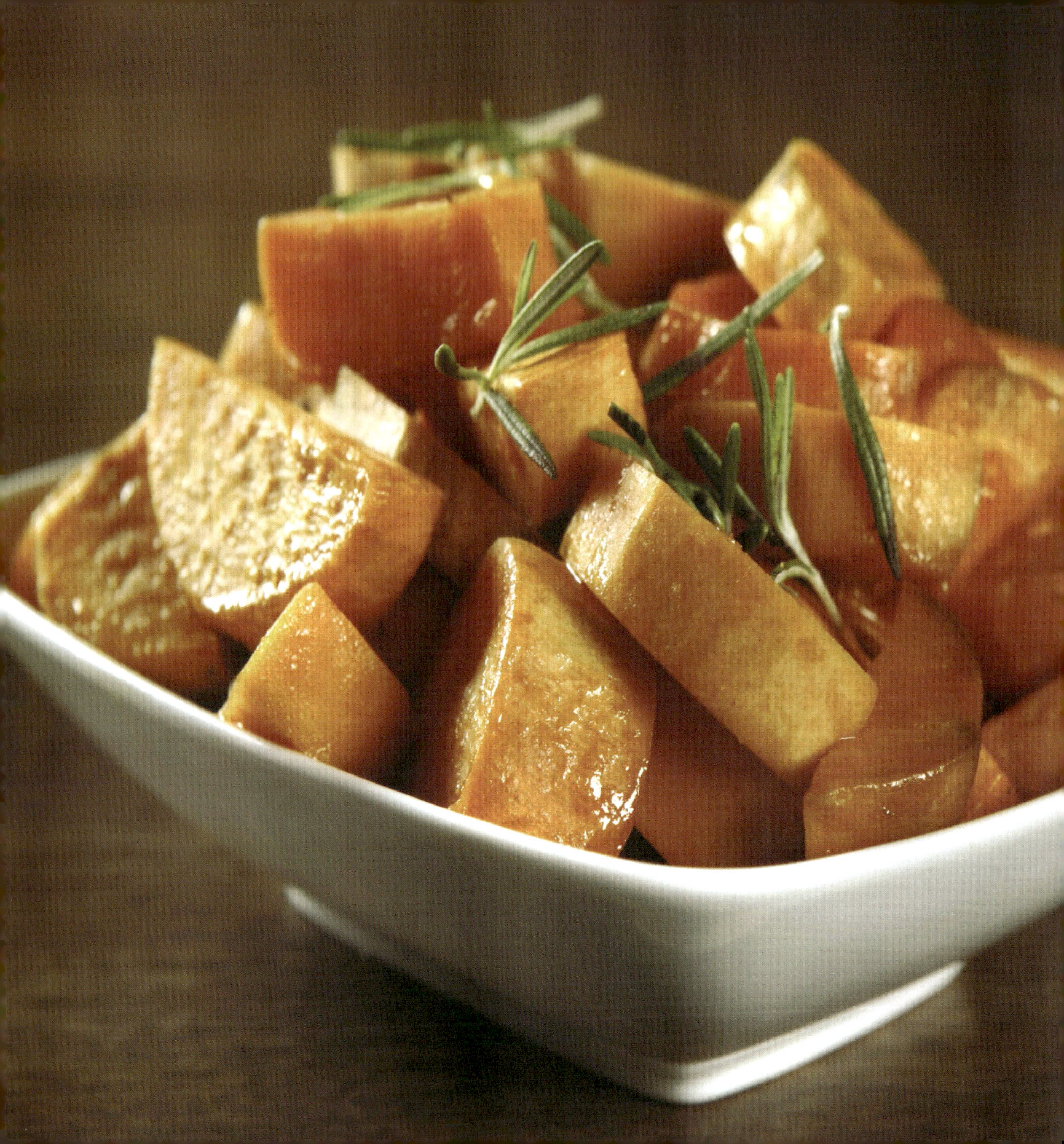

Roasted Sweet Potatoes with Fall Spices

6 sweet potatoes, peeled and quartered

¼ cup olive oil

Fall Spices

½ tbs. cinnamon

¼ tbs. nutmeg

¼ tsp. all-spice

Instructions

Preheat oven to 400 degrees. Rinse potatoes and dry with a paper towel. Peel and cut potatoes in half, then into quarters. Place cut potatoes on a baking sheet. Season with cinnamon, nutmeg, and all-spice. Pour olive oil on potatoes. Toss to ensure potatoes are evenly coated with fall spices and olive oil. Place in oven for 30-45 minutes until potatoes are brown. Flip halfway through cooking time to ensure even browning. Test doneness by piercing the potatoes in the center with a sharp knife. If the knife goes through easily, then they are done.

Tip: To add a different style to this dish, you can cut the sweet potatoes lengthwise to create sweet potatoes fries. Ensure that all potatoes are the same thickness so that they will cook evenly. Finish the sweet potatoes off with additional fall seasoning once done.

Serving Size: 4

Brown Rice Pilaf

4 servings Uncle Ben's Fast & Natural instant brown rice, whole grain

2 tbs. olive oil

1 large shallot, diced

Salt and pepper to taste

Instructions

Prepare rice according to package directions. Peel and chop shallot. In a large skillet heat olive oil on medium heat and sauté shallots until tender. Add prepared rice to skillet. Add salt and pepper to taste.

Tip: This is a great side dish with grilled chicken or fish after the Daniel Fast.

Serving Size: 4

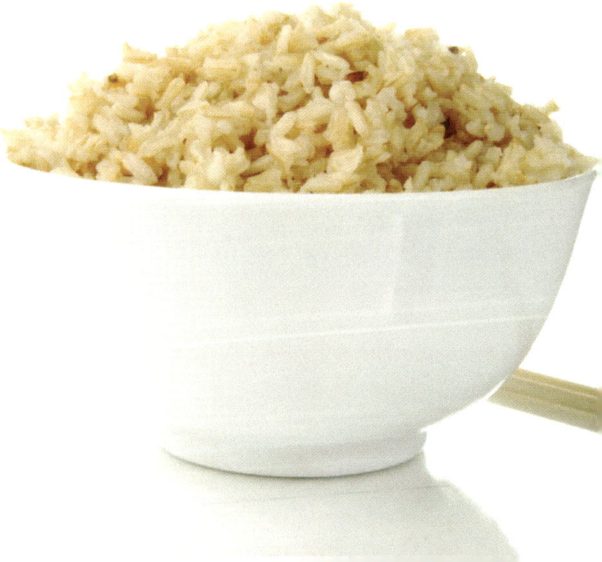

Sauté Cabbage with Bell Peppers

1 large head cabbage, cubed

1 yellow bell pepper, diced

1 red bell pepper, diced

½ cup water

½ tsp. black pepper

2 tbs. olive oil

1 orange bell pepper, diced

1 large onion, minced

1 tbs. white vinegar

½ tsp. kosher salt

Instructions

Cut cabbage in half. Remove core and slice cabbage halves diagonally; rotate a quarter turn and slice lengthwise. This will create small cubes of cabbage. Remove seeds from bell peppers and dice the peppers, then prepare onion as instructed. In a large frying pan with a lid add olive oil; sauté onion and bell peppers on medium-high heat until tender. Add cabbage to mixture and sauté for 1-2 minutes. Add water to pan and allow cabbage to steam for approximately 10-15 minutes or until tender. When cabbage is tender add the pepper, salt, and vinegar to taste.

Tip: For enhanced flavor after the Daniel Fast you can add 1 tablespoon of sugar for a more robust flavor.

Serving Size: 8

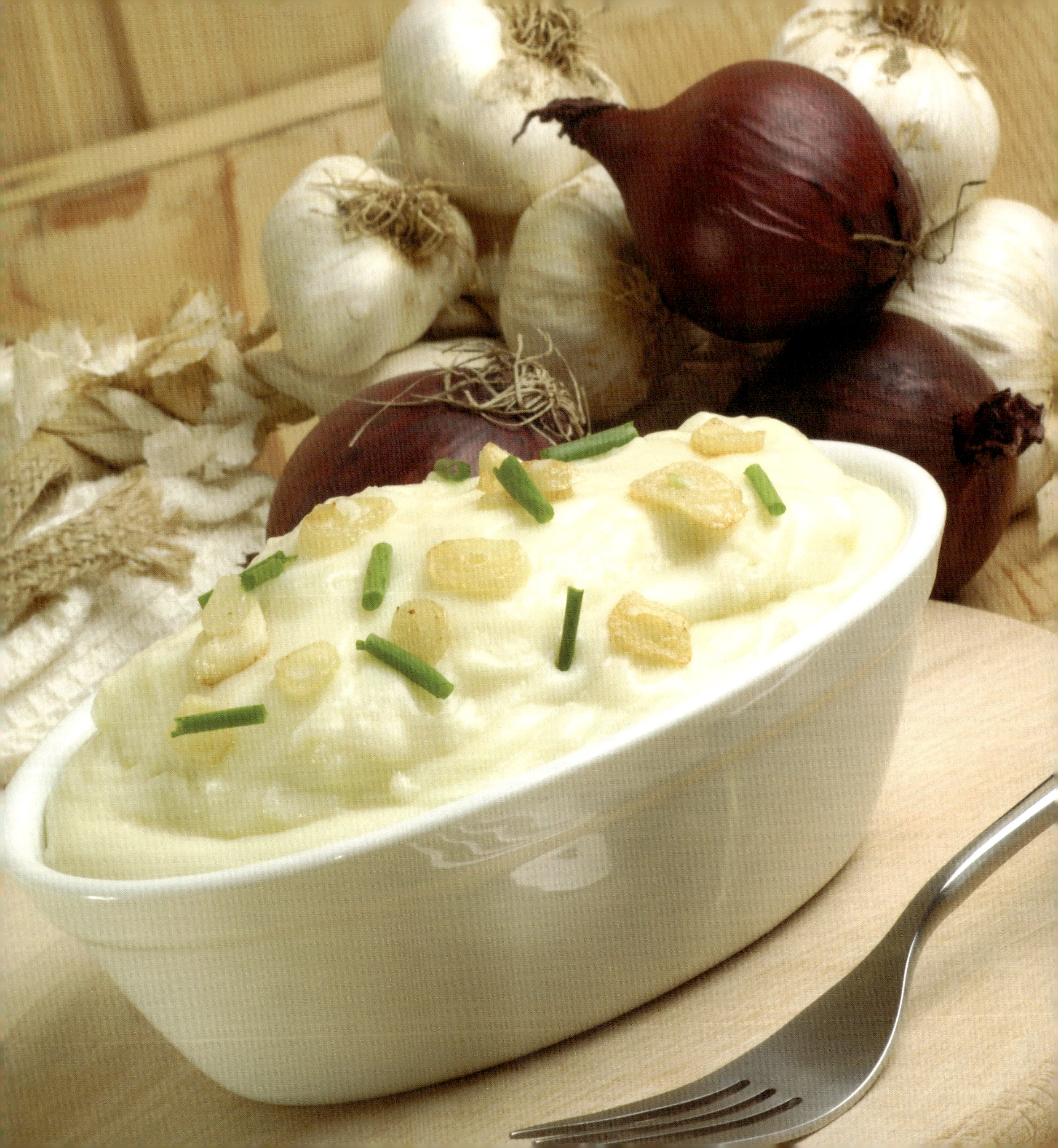

Garlic Smashed Potatoes

6 cups water	6 medium red skin potatoes, quartered
2 tsp. kosher salt	⅓ cup garlic-infused olive oil (see instructions on page 55)
½ tsp. black pepper	8-10 roasted garlic bulbs (see instructions on page 57)

Instructions

Clean and rinse potatoes. Cut potatoes into quarters and place in a large pot and cover with water. Add ½ teaspoon of salt to water and bring to a rapid boil for approximately 25 minutes or until potatoes are tender. Drain potatoes and place in a mixing bowl.

Add the roasted garlic cloves, garlic-infused olive oil, remaining salt and pepper to potatoes. Use a large steel serving spoon to smash potatoes by cutting them with the side of the spoon against the side of the bowl. Adjust salt and pepper to preferred taste if desired.

Tip: After the Daniel Fast you can use this recipe as a side dish for many meal. Add 2 tablespoons unsalted butter and ½ cup sour cream for an enhanced flavor.

Serving Size: 6

Sautéed Spinach with Garlic

1 pkg. fresh baby spinach

½ tsp. kosher salt

2 tbs. olive oil

2 garlic bulbs, thinly sliced

¼ tsp. black pepper

Instructions

In a large skillet add olive oil and heat on medium-high. Peel garlic and slice into thin slices. Add garlic to hot oil to allow garlic to penetrate the oil. Add the baby spinach and cook for 1-2 minutes or until spinach is wilted. Add salt and pepper to taste.

Tip: You can use garlic infused oil (see page 55) with this recipe to enhance the garlic flavor.

Serving Size: 4

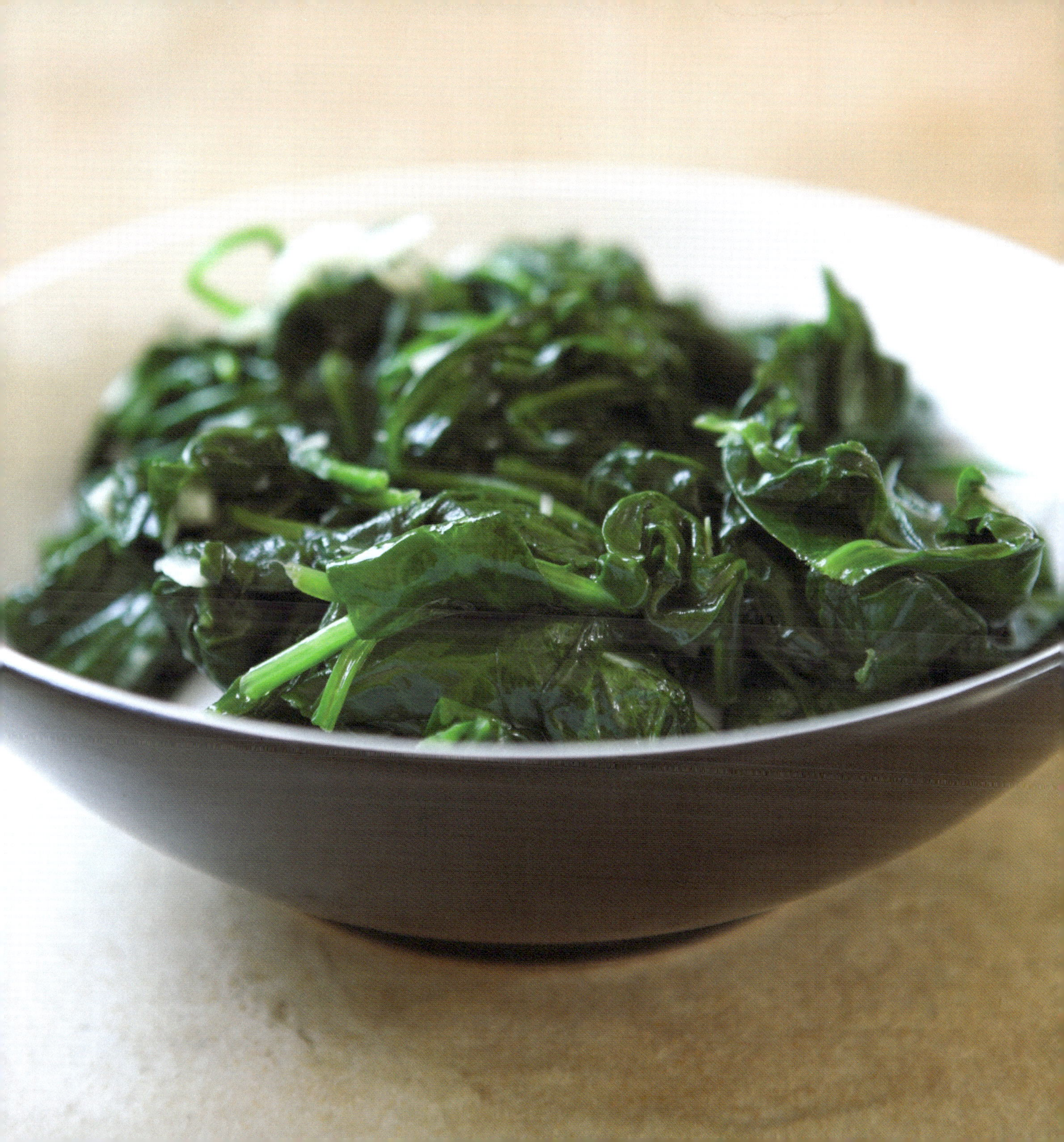

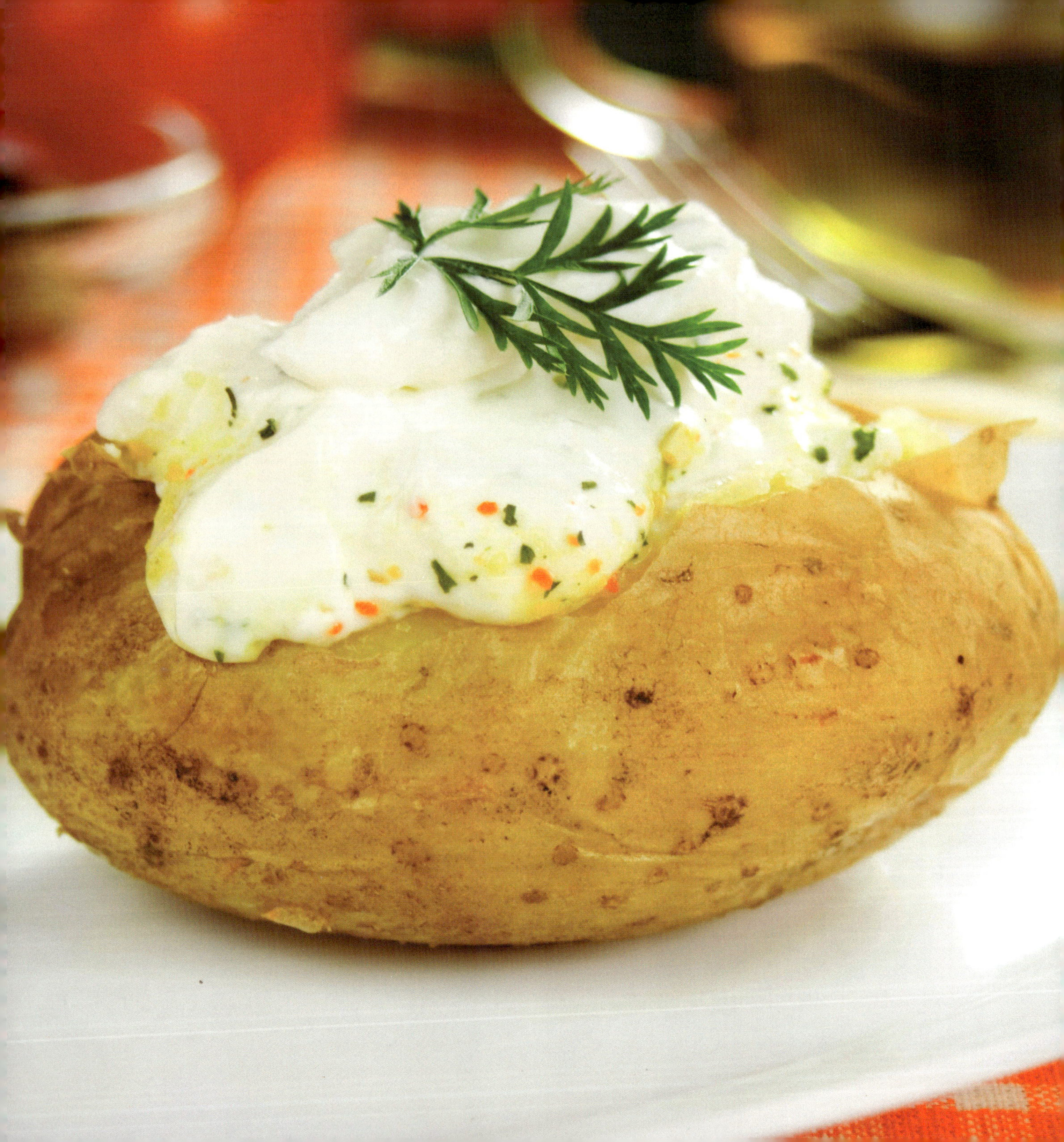

Baked Potato with Tofu Sour Cream & Chives

2 large russet potatoes

½ tsp. chives, chopped

⅓ cup kosher salt

½ cup tofu sour cream (as prepared on page 46)

Instructions

Preheat oven to 400 degrees. Wash the potatoes to remove dirt. Roll wet potatoes in kosher salt and place in middle of top oven rack. You may want to put a baking sheet on the rack under the potatoes to catch the salt if it falls off. Bake potatoes in oven for approximately 1 hour or until soft. When done, wrap in aluminum foil until ready to serve. Remove aluminum foil and cut open potatoes. Add tofu sour cream, salt, pepper, and chives to taste. Serve and enjoy.

Tip: You can prepare the potatoes 30 minutes before serving to save time. When potatoes are done, turn off the oven, wrap potatoes in aluminum foil, and place them back in the oven to retain warmth until serving dinner.

Serving Size: 2

Potato Cakes

4 large russet potatoes, peeled and grated

1 tsp. kosher salt

⅓ cup olive oil

½ tsp. black pepper

Instructions

Wash and peel potatoes. Use a box grater or mandolin slicer to grate potatoes into medium shreds. Place shredded potatoes in water to keep them from turning brown. In a large skillet add olive oil and heat over medium heat. Drain potatoes and add salt and pepper. Layer the shredded potatoes in small, round batches in the oil, ensuring that they are all connected—you should not be able to see the bottom of the pan. You can typically fit 4-5 small potato cakes in a large skillet. Allow potatoes to brown in oil for 2-3 minutes until they stick together and are lightly browned on one side. Flip the cakes over with a spatula and brown the other side. If you turn them over and they fall apart, they are not done. Turn back over and allow to brown on the original side for an additional 1-2 minutes, then flip over to brown the other side. Once browned on both sides remove from oil and place on a dry towel to remove excess oil. Finish by seasoning with additional salt and pepper to taste.

Tip: If you have a mandolin slicer use the julienne setting for thinly sliced shreds. This works perfectly and is great if you want to make one large potato cake instead of several smaller ones.

Serving Size: 8

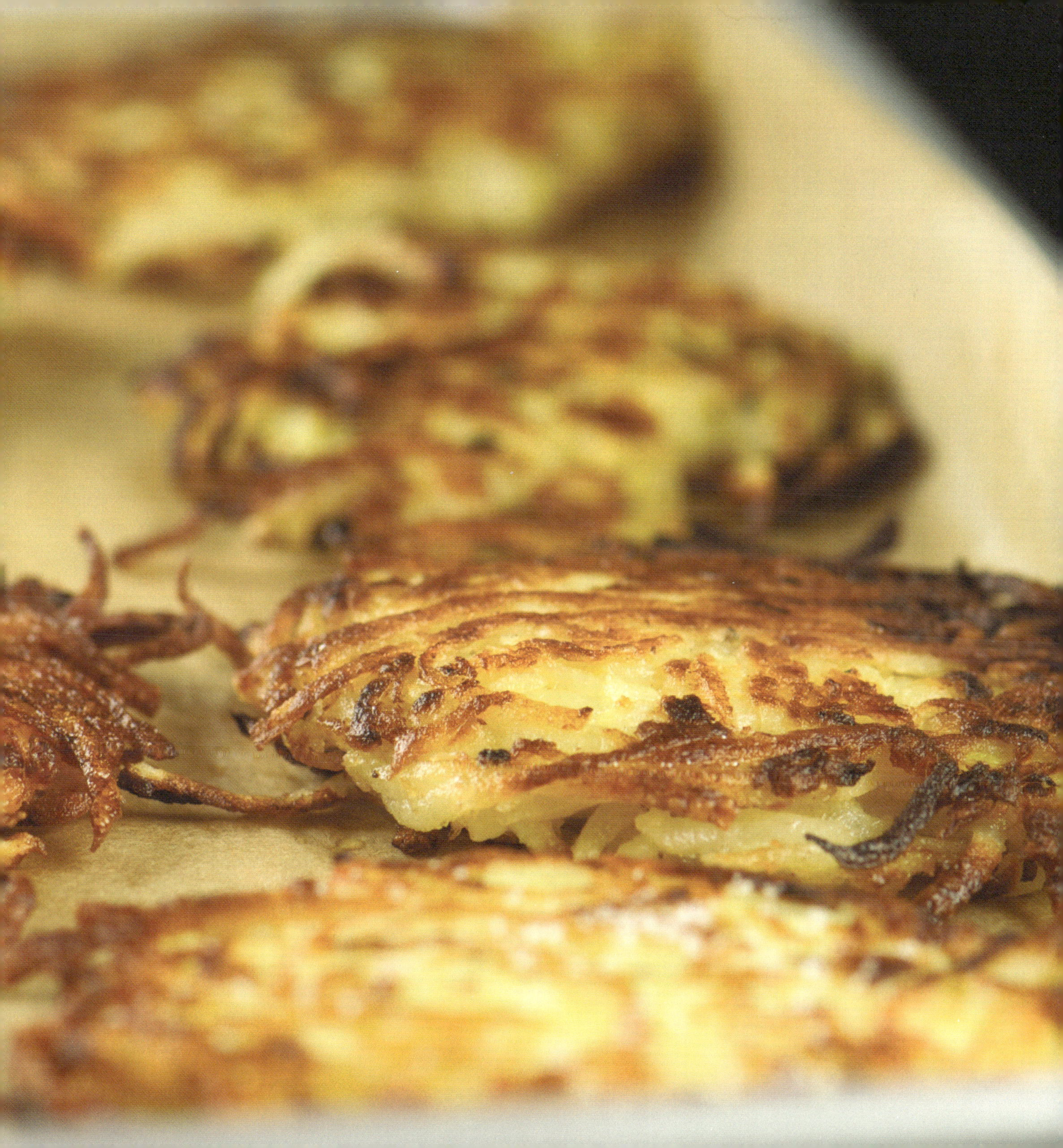

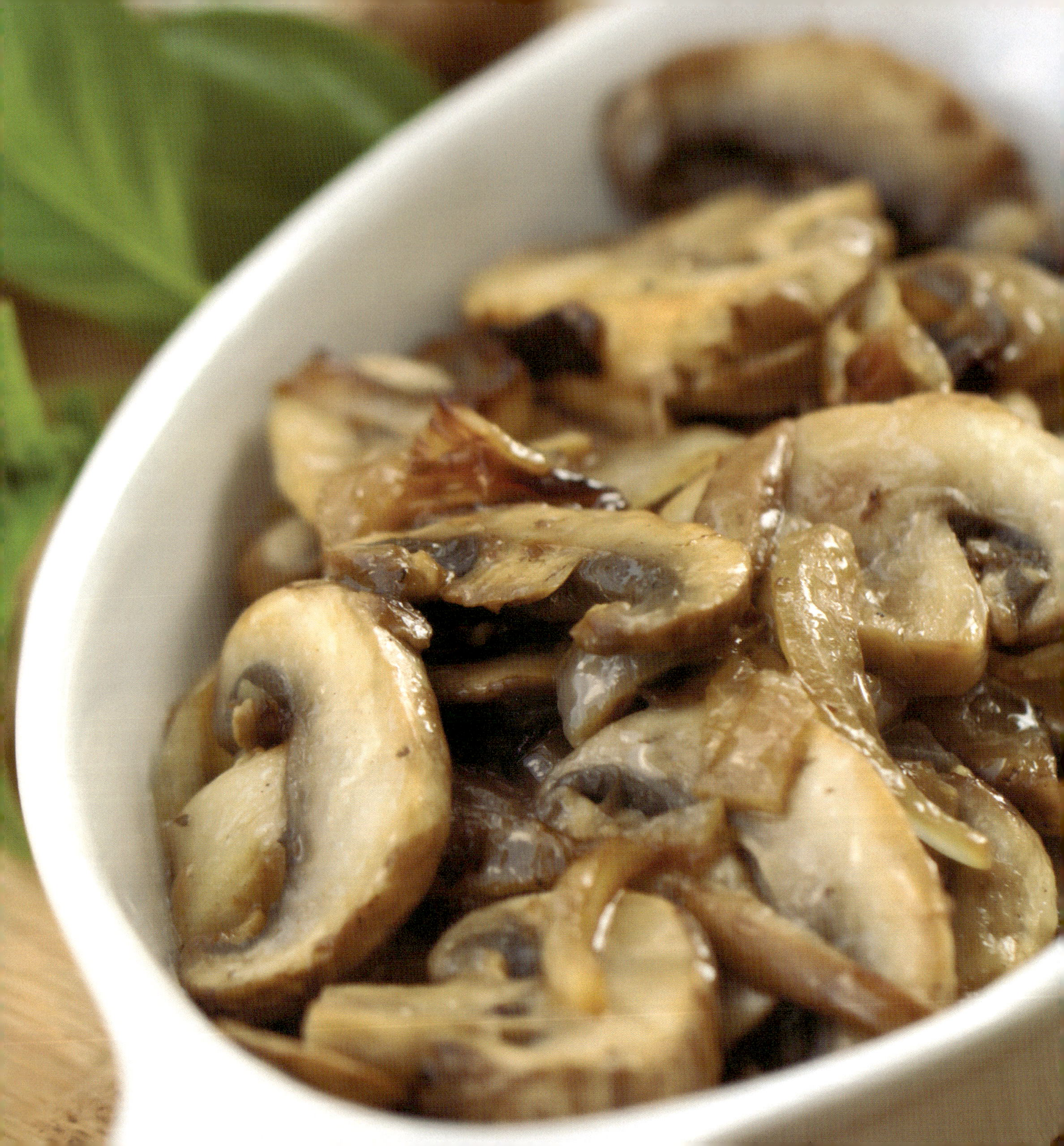

Sautéed Mushrooms & Onions

1 pint baby bella mushrooms, whole or sliced

3 garlic cloves, minced

½ tsp. black pepper

1 tbs. sugar (optional post Daniel Fast)

1 large sweet onion, peeled and sliced

1 tsp. kosher salt

¼ cup olive oil

Instructions

Prepare onions and garlic as instructed above and set aside until later. In a large skillet heat olive oil on medium-low heat. Add onion, mushrooms, salt, and pepper and cook until onions becomes translucent and starts to caramelize or brown. This will take approximately 10-15 minutes. Stir the mixture frequently to ensure onions and mushrooms do not burn. Once the onions are translucent and caramelized, add minced garlic and cook 2-3 minutes to remove the raw garlic taste. You may need to add additional salt and pepper to taste.

Tip: The key to having perfectly caramelized onions is to cook them over low-medium heat and toss occasionally to ensure even cooking, making sure the onions do not burn. Once the Daniel Fast is over, you can add 1 tablespoon of sugar, which will help the onions caramelize evenly.

Serving Size: 2

Homemade Sweet Potato Fries

6 sweet potatoes	¼ cup olive oil

Fall Spices

½ tbs. cinnamon	¼ tbs. nutmeg
¼ tsp. all-spice	1 tbs. sugar (optional after fast is over)

Instructions

Preheat oven to 400 degrees. Rinse potatoes and dry with a paper towel. Peel skin and cut potatoes in half, and then into even, lengthwise strips. Cut potatoes will resemble French fries. In a large bowl toss sweet potato fries with olive oil to ensure all cut edges are coated. Place sweet potato fries evenly on baking sheets and place in oven for 30-45 minutes or until potatoes are tender and slightly brown. Toss potatoes halfway through to ensure even browning. Test doneness by piercing potatoes in the center with a sharp knife. If the knife goes through easily, they are done. Remove from oven and while the sweet potato fries are still hot; toss in a large bowl with fall spices.

Serving Size: 4

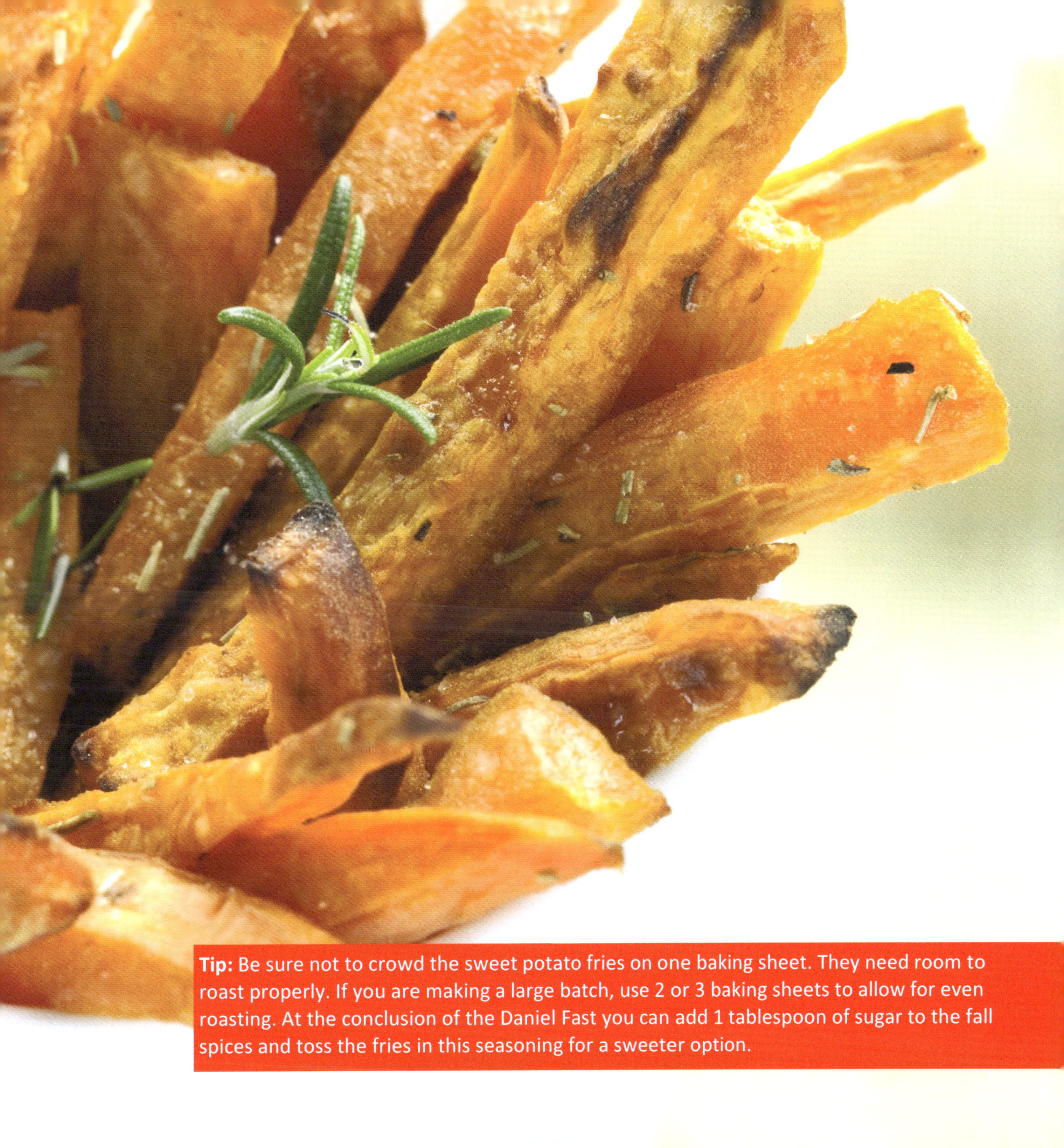

Tip: Be sure not to crowd the sweet potato fries on one baking sheet. They need room to roast properly. If you are making a large batch, use 2 or 3 baking sheets to allow for even roasting. At the conclusion of the Daniel Fast you can add 1 tablespoon of sugar to the fall spices and toss the fries in this seasoning for a sweeter option.

Potato & Onions

1 large sweet onion, julienned

½ tsp. salt

½ cup water

6 russet or red skin potatoes, ¼ inch slices

¼ tsp. black pepper

¼ cup olive oil plus additional 2 tbs.

Instructions

Wash, peel, and slice potatoes into ¼ inch rounds. Peel and julienne onions. Combine onions and potatoes in a large frying pan. Add 2 tablespoons of olive oil. Then add salt and pepper. Cook onions until they become translucent and potatoes until they begin to brown. Add water, cover pan, and turn on medium-high heat, allowing the potatoes and onions to steam and become tender. You will need to watch the potatoes and turn them over periodically through this process to allow for even baking.

When the potatoes and onions are tender and the water has evaporated from the pan, add the olive oil to bottom of pan, allowing the potatoes to lightly brown. Add additional salt and pepper to taste.

Tip: This is a great dish to have for breakfast post Daniel Fast.

Serving Size: 6

Roasted Asparagus

1 bunch green asparagus

1 tbs. kosher salt

¼ cup olive oil

½ tbs. black pepper

Instructions

Preheat oven to 400 degrees. Place asparagus on cutting board and cut off woody stems; this is typically about 1 inch of the bottom. Align cut asparagus on a baking sheet in an even row. Add salt and pepper and toss to make sure asparagus is evenly seasoned. Drizzle olive oil and toss to make sure asparagus is evenly coated. Roast 15-20 minutes or until tender. You can shake the pan to roll the asparagus over halfway through the cooking process so that it browns evenly.

Tip: This is a great side dish for any meal.

Serving Size: 4

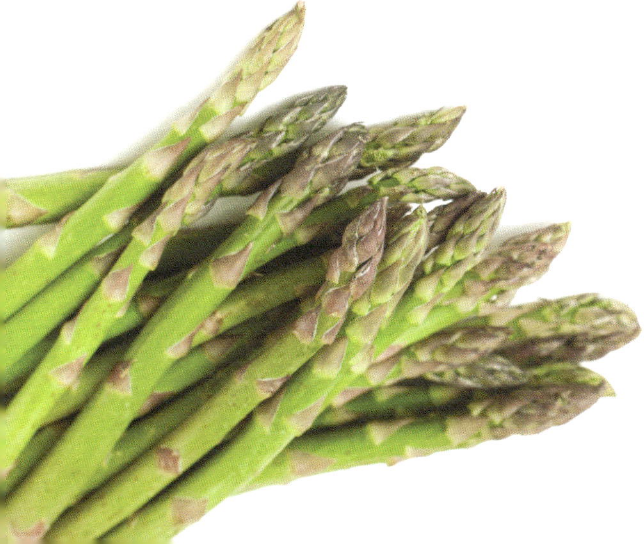

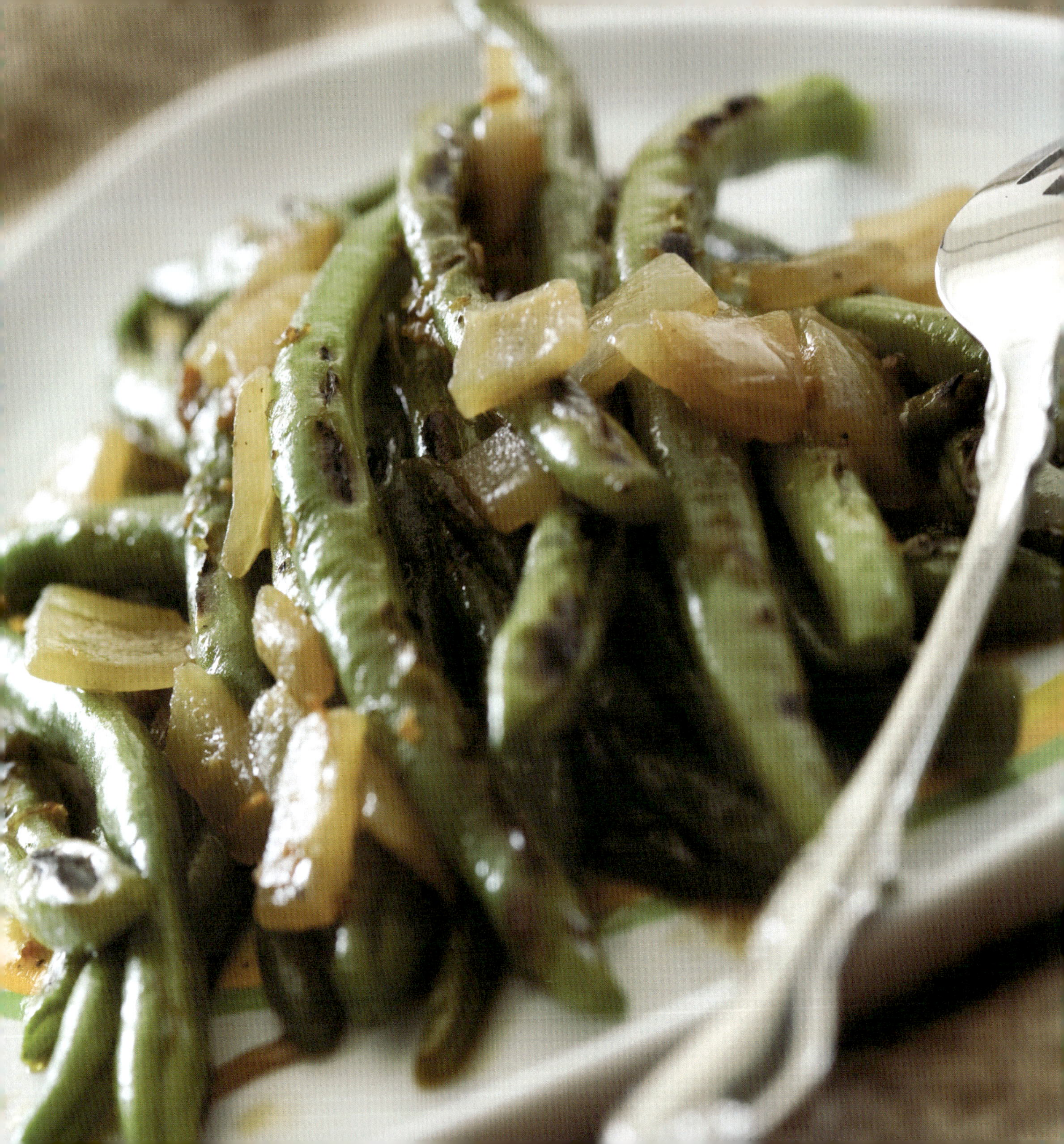

Sautéed Green Beans with Onions

3 quarts water

2 medium sweet onions, julienned

4 tbs. balsamic vinegar

½ tsp. black pepper

1 ½ lbs. fresh green beans

3 tbs. olive oil

1 tsp. kosher salt plus 1 tbs.

Instructions

Wash green beans in cold water. Break off both ends, and discard. Snap remaining beans in half and place in a large bowl. In a large stockpot bring water to a boil and add 1 tablespoon of salt. Add the prepared green beans to boiling water and cook 8-10 minutes or until tender. Drain green beans and place in a bowl of ice water to stop the cooking process.

In a large skillet add 2 tablespoons of olive oil and sauté onions over medium-high heat until translucent and caramelized. Drain green beans and add to onions. Sauté for 2-3 minutes. Remove green beans from heat and add remaining salt, pepper, and balsamic vinegar to taste.

Tip: You may need to add 1 tablespoon of additional olive oil to the skillet when you add the green beans to ensure that they do not stick or burn. You may also need to add additional salt and pepper to taste.

Serving Size: 6

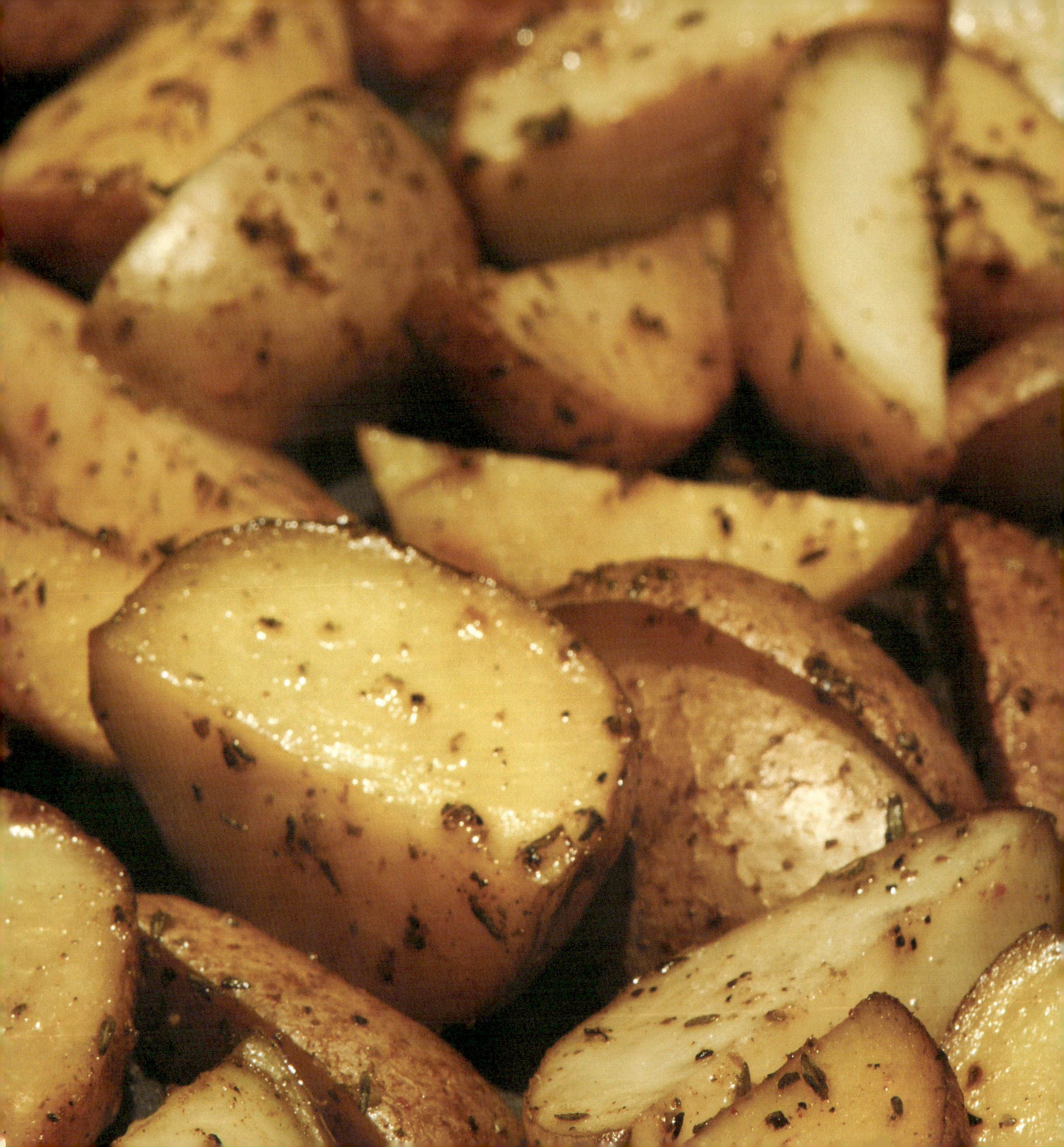

Roasted Red Skin Potatoes

6 red skin potatoes, quartered

1 tbs. kosher salt

⅓ cup olive oil

½ tbs. black pepper

Instructions

Preheat oven to 400 degrees. Rinse potatoes and dry with a paper towel. Cut potatoes in half, then into quarters. Place cut potatoes on a baking sheet and season with salt and pepper. Pour on olive oil and toss to ensure potatoes are evenly coated. Place in oven for 30-45 minutes until potatoes are brown. Flip potatoes with a spatula halfway through cooking time to ensure even browning. Test doneness by piercing the center of potatoes with a sharp knife. If the knife goes through easily, then they are done.

Tip: If you have a convection roast setting on your oven, you can use it to reduce the cooking time by 10 minutes.

Serving Size: 4

I will give you a new heart and put a new spirit within you; I will take the heart of stone out of your flesh and give you a heart of flesh. I will put My Spirit within you and cause you to walk in My statutes, and you will keep My judgments and do them. Ezekiel 36:26-27

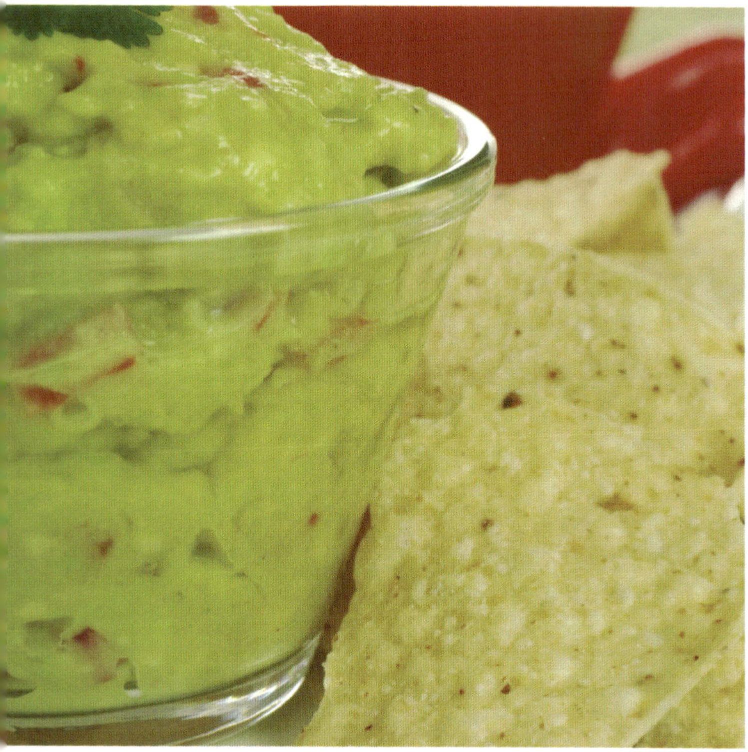

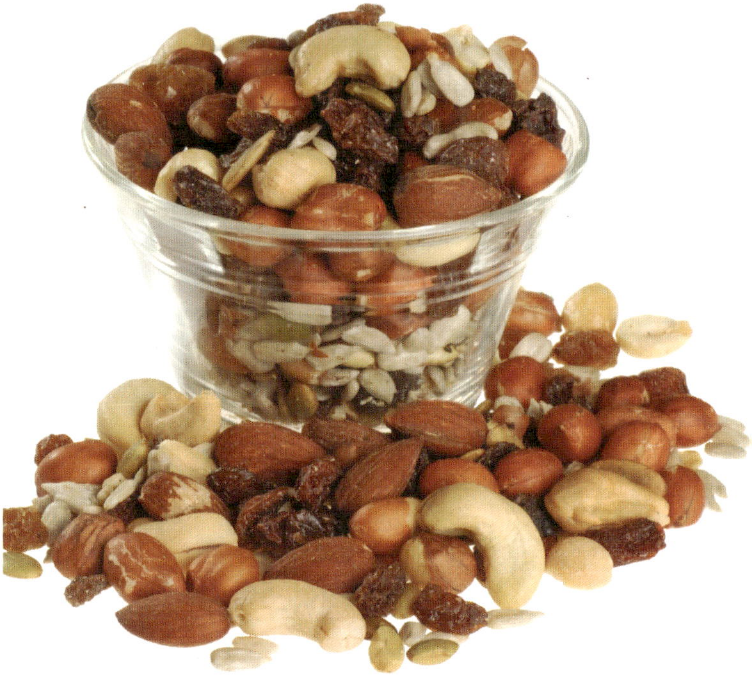

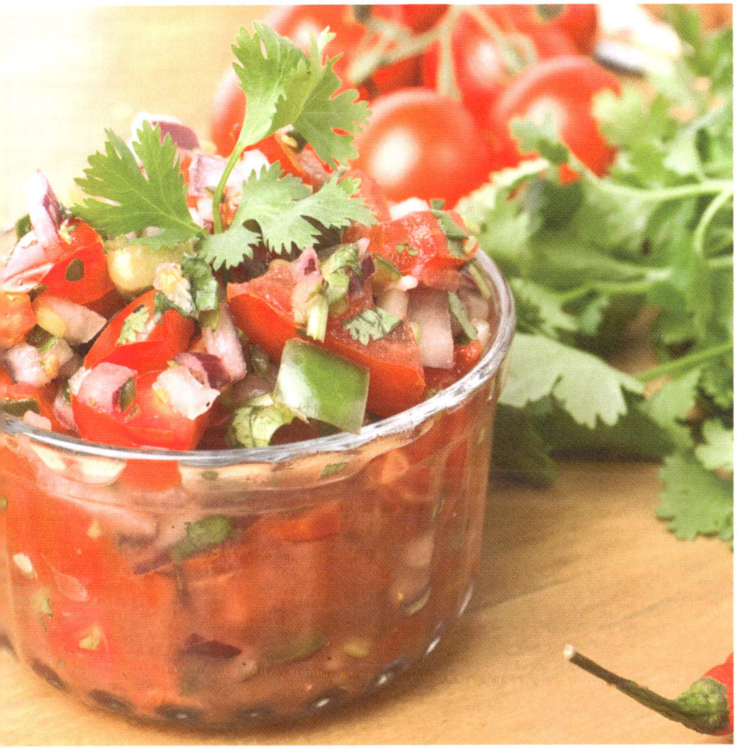

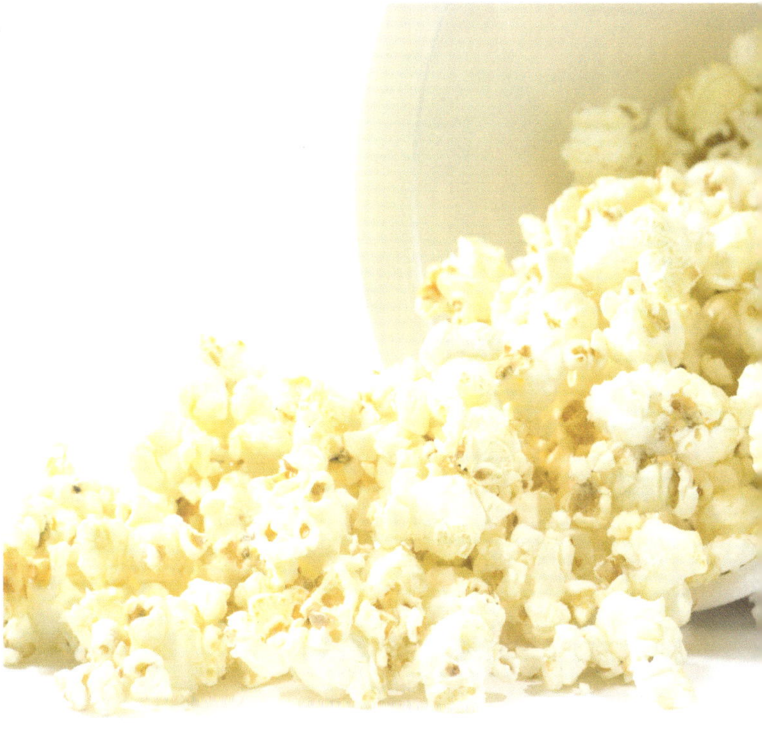

Snacks

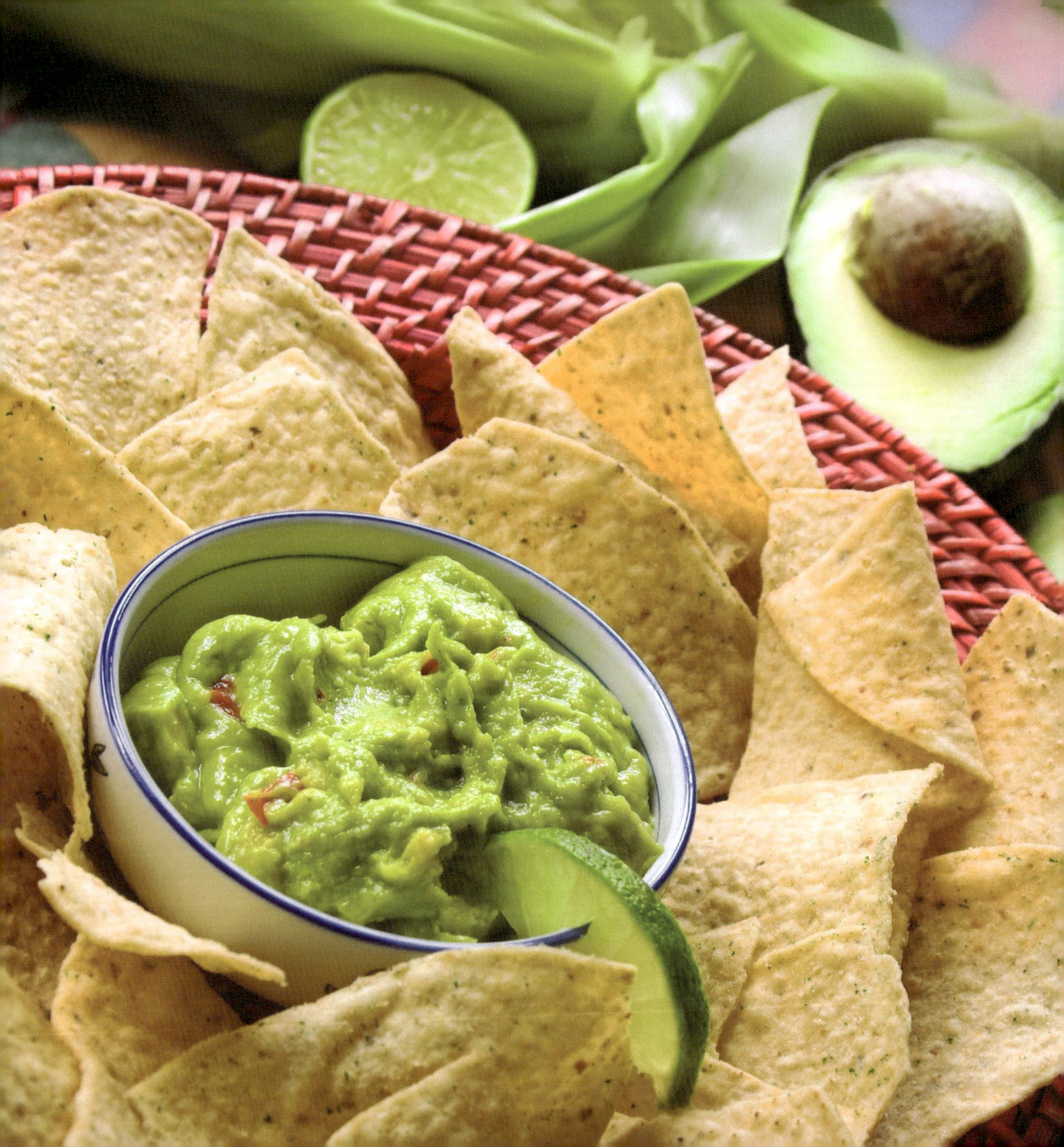

Guacamole with Baked Tortilla Chips

2 ripe Haas avocados

1 large garlic clove (minced)

Salt & pepper to taste

1 vine-ripened tomato, seeded

1 small shallot, minced

¼ cup lime juice

4-5 dashes of hot sauce (optional)

Instructions

Cut avocado in half, remove pit, and scoop flesh away from skin. Place in a large bowl and add lime juice immediately to avoid browning. Add shallots, garlic, and tomatoes as instructed. Smash avocado with the back of a fork until the desired texture is reached. Add salt, pepper, and hot sauce to taste.

Tip: Look for 100% baked corn chips to enjoy with guacamole. If you prefer, you can also use this recipe as a spread for vegetable wraps, or enjoy it in a salad.

Serving Size: 4

Homemade Popcorn

⅓ cup corn kernels

⅓ cup peanut oil

1 large heavy bottom pot with lid

Instructions

Combine oil and corn kernels in a pot with a lid and place on burner. Heat on medium-high for 10 minutes. Shake the pot throughout the cooking process to ensure even popping. You will hear the popcorn pop throughout the cooking process. When popping stops, the popcorn is done. Turn heat off and remove lid to allow popcorn to cool. Add seasoning for added flavor.

Using the right seasonings will make your popcorn even more enjoyable! Use one of the seasoning options below to add an extra flare to your snack.

- Option #1: Add 2 tsp. garlic powder with 1 tsp. kosher salt
- Option #2: Use 2 tsp. season salt with ¼ tsp. black pepper
- Option #3: 1 tsp. garlic powder with 1 tsp. kosher salt and ¼ tsp. black pepper

Tip: This recipe is kid friendly and can be a great way to get kids involved in your Daniel Fast, while providing everyone with a healthy treat. But please note, popcorn is considered a choking hazard for children under age 3.

Serving Size: 6

Snack Trail Mix

½ cup raisins

½ cup dried cranberries

¼ cup roasted cashews

¼ tsp. cinnamon

⅔ cup dried banana chips

¼ cup roasted almonds

⅔ cup toasted coconut

½ cup dried papaya, diced

Instructions

Preheat oven to 400 degrees. Combine almonds, cashews, and coconut on an ungreased baking sheet. Sprinkle cinnamon over mixture evenly. Roast in oven for 10-15 minutes. Remove from oven and allow to cool completely; place in a large bowl. Add raisins, dried banana chips, papaya and dried cranberries to the mixture.

Tip: This all-natural mix is naturally sweet and a great snack. Place individually-sized portions in small sandwich bags for a quick, portable snack. If you make a large batch, house in an air-tight container to retain freshness.

Serving Size: 6

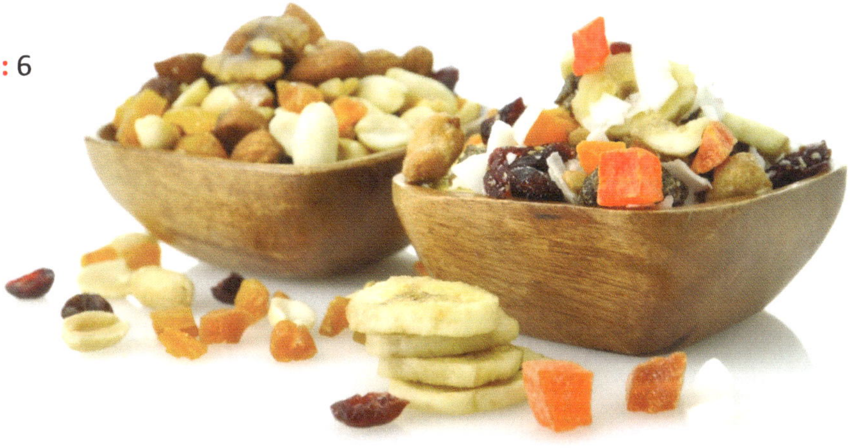

Black Bean & Corn Salsa

1 pkg. frozen corn

2 garlic cloves, minced

1 tbs. olive oil

1 lime, juiced

1 poblano pepper, seeded and diced

4 roma tomatoes, seeded and diced

½ tsp. kosher salt

¼ tsp. black pepper

1 can Goya black beans, drained and rinsed (15.5 oz.)

1 jalapeño pepper, seeded and chopped into small pieces

Instructions

Preheat oven to 400 degrees. Line a baking sheet with aluminum foil, pour oil in hand, and rub oil on poblano pepper, jalapeño pepper, and tomatoes. Place all vegetables on baking sheet and add frozen corn. Roast vegetables in oven for 30-35 minutes. Remove from oven and allow vegetables to cool slightly. Remove charred skin from peppers and prepare each vegetable according to instructions. In a large mixing bowl combine roasted vegetables, garlic, salt, and pepper. Drain and rinse black beans in cool water and add to vegetable mixture. Squeeze lime juice over mixture and enjoy on a baked corn tortilla.

Tip: This is a great topping that can go on vegetables, chicken, or fish. If you prefer a hotter salsa you can chop the jalapeño and poblano peppers whole without removing the seeds or veins.

Serving Size: 4

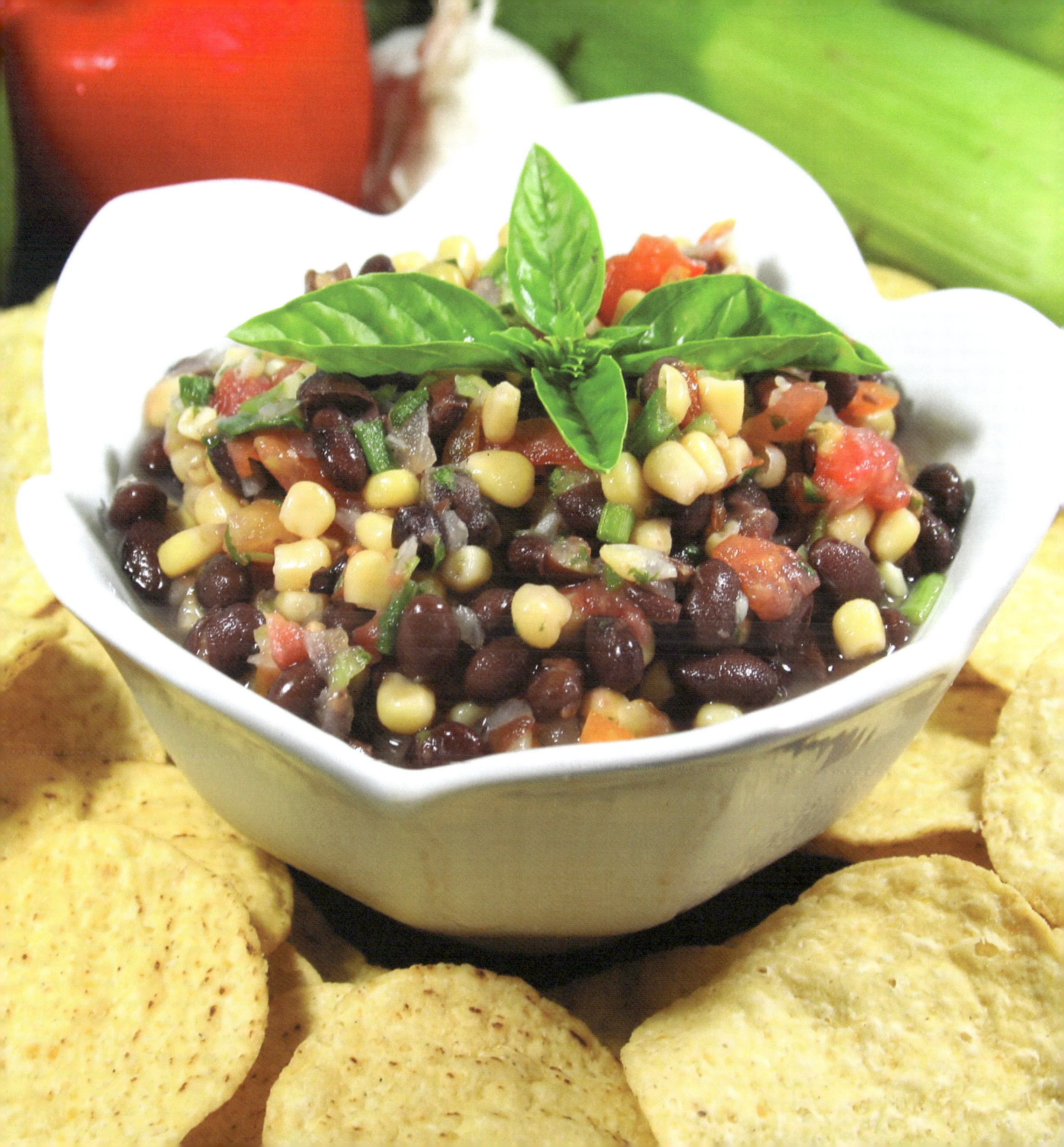

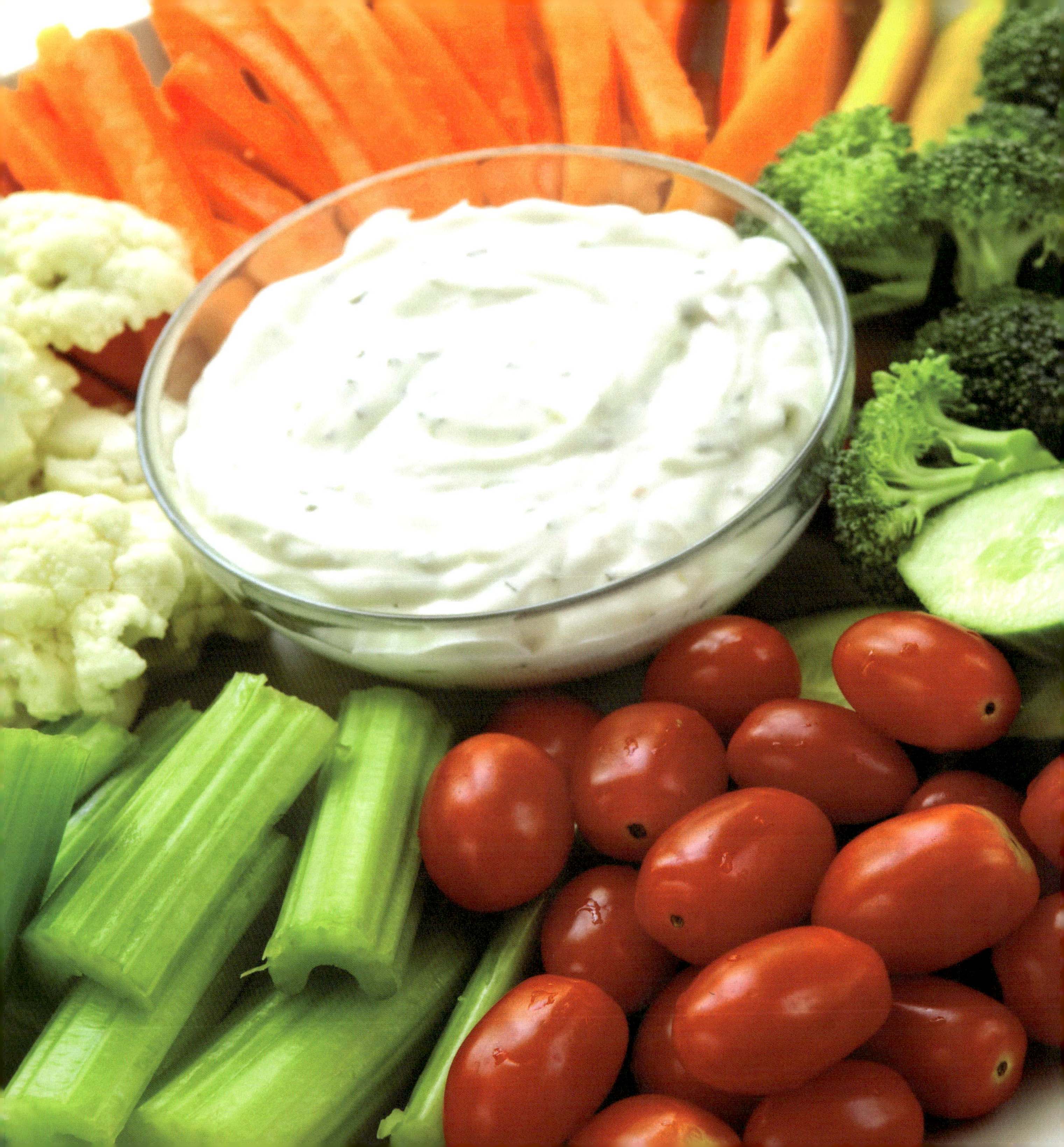

Vegetable Crudités with French Onion Dip

1 bunch broccoli

1 small pack of baby carrots

1 pint grape tomatoes

1 orange bell pepper

1 head cauliflower

1 large cucumber, sliced

1 yellow bell pepper

4 celery stalks

Instructions

Cut vegetables into bite-sized pieces. Place a dip service bowl in the middle of platter. Arrange each vegetable by type on the platter. Fill the bowl with the French onion dip and serve.

Tips: Use the instructions on page 46 to create the French onion dip.

Serving Size: 6

Now to Him who is able to do exceedingly abundantly above all that we ask or think, according to the power that works in us, to Him be glory in the church by Christ Jesus to all generations, forever and ever. Amen. Ephesians 3:20-21

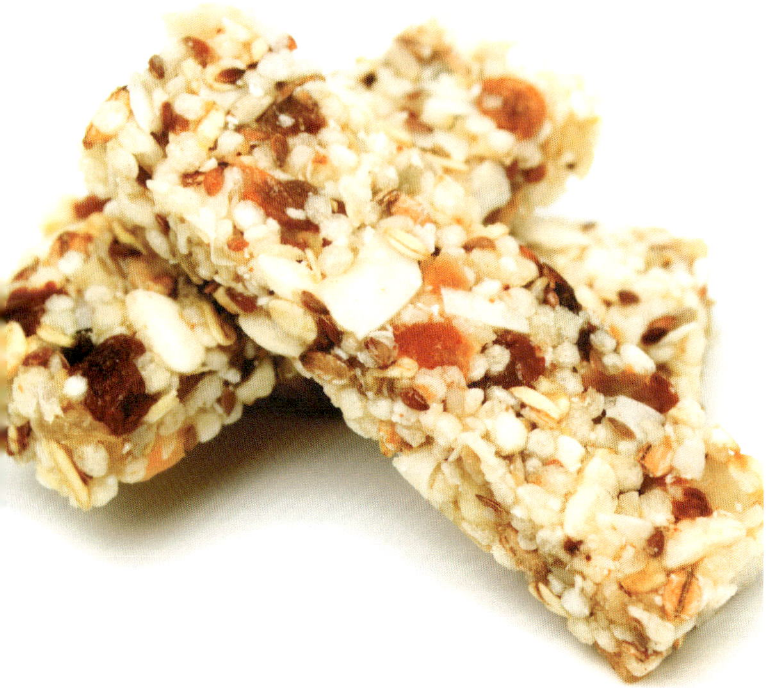

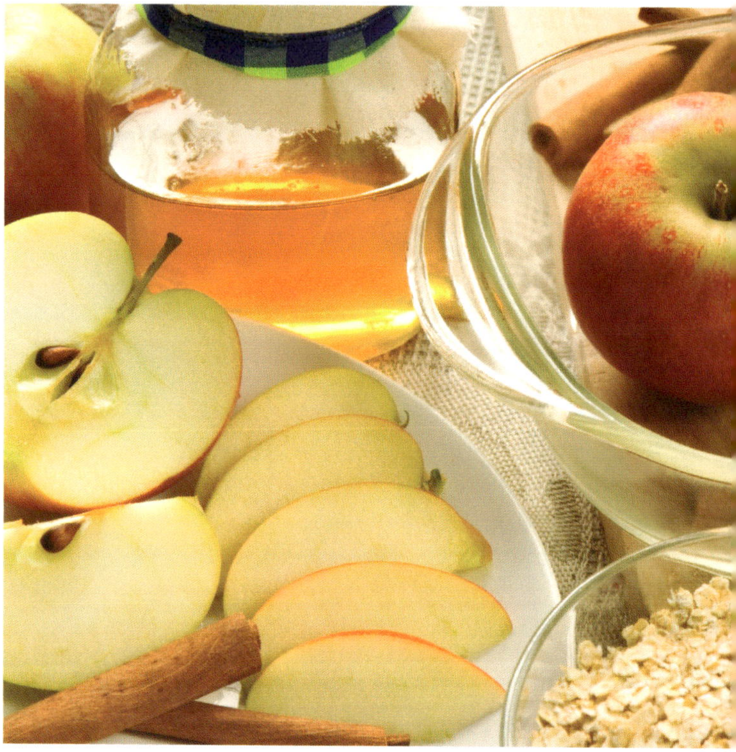

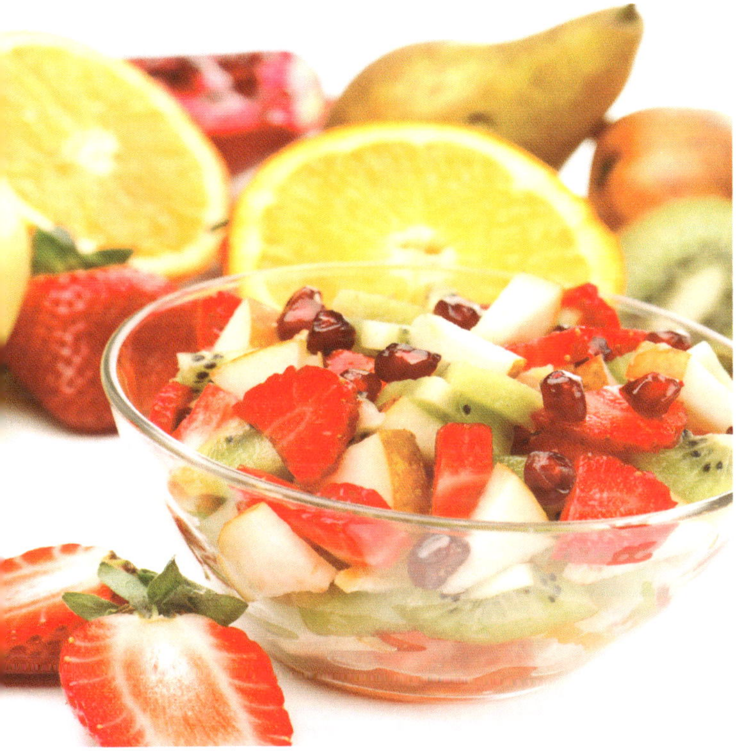

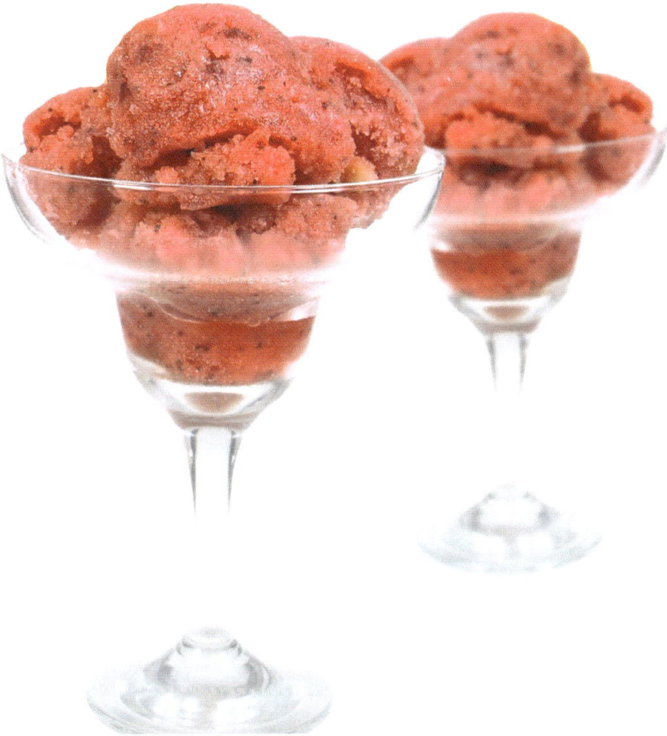

Desserts

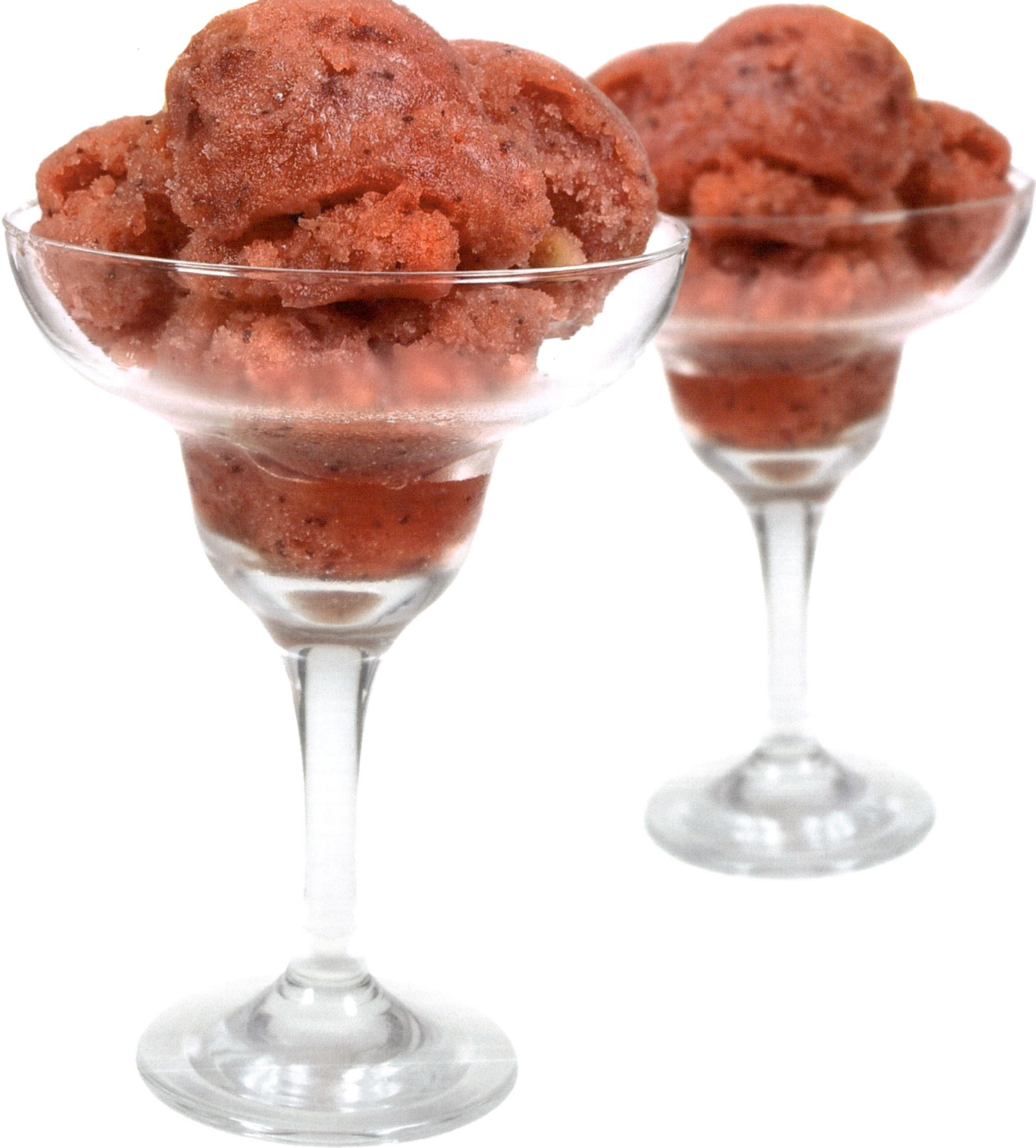

Strawberry Lime Sorbet

1 ½ cups Blue Mountain agave nectar

2 cups fresh strawberries, stems removed

2 cups cold water

1 tbs. lime zest

Instructions

Combine all ingredients into a blender. Blend until smooth and a froth forms on the top. Pour mixture into a freezer-proof bowl and place in freezer overnight (or until solid). Scoop sorbet out with ice cream scoop and serve in an ice cream sundae glass. Garnish with a strawberry on the rim.

Tip: Agave nectar is an all-natural sweetener substitute. If your Daniel Fast prohibits sugar, I recommend making this at the conclusion of your Daniel Fast experience. You may also substitute other fruit (pineapples, mangos, blueberries) for a different sorbet flavor.

Serving Size: 8

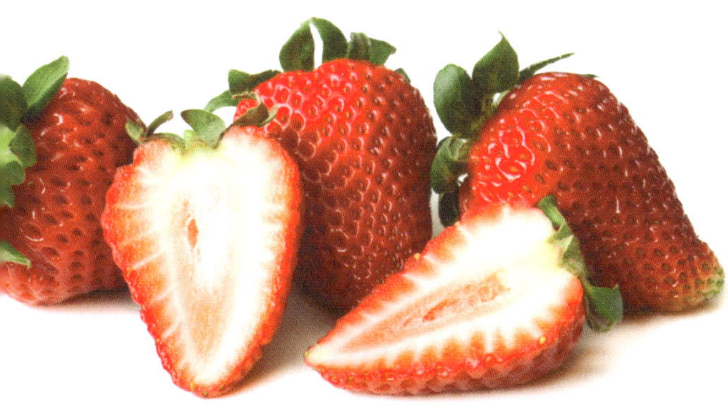

Roasted Apple with Oatmeal & Dried Cranberries

2 Granny Smith apples

½ cup dried cran-raisins

½ tsp. nutmeg

¼ cup 100% apple juice

½ cup old fashioned rolled oats

½ tsp. cinnamon

¼ tsp. all-spice

Instructions

Preheat oven to 375 degrees. Slice apple in half and remove the core; place apples cut side up in a small ovenproof casserole dish. In a small bowl combine cinnamon, nutmeg, and all-spice. Take half of spice mixture and mix with oats and cran-raisins in another bowl. Place a spoonful of the mixture into core of apple. Sprinkle remaining spices on cut surface of apple. Pour apple juice in the bottom of pan. Bake apples for 30-45 minutes or until soft, and until the oatmeal mixture is light brown.

Tip: Once your Daniel Fast is over, add ¼ cup of sugar to cinnamon, nutmeg, and all-spice mixture and sprinkle on cut surface of apples.

Serving Size: 2

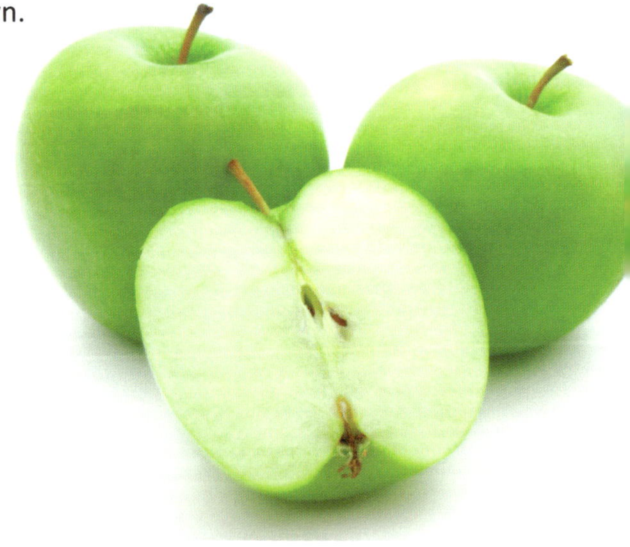

Fruit Salad

1 golden pineapple, diced

1 honeydew melon, diced

1 kiwi, bite-sized pieces

1 cantaloupe, diced

1 pint strawberries, quartered

¼ cup apple or orange juice

Instructions

Cut off top and bottom of pineapple, then stand upright and remove outer skin. Cut the pineapple lengthwise and remove the inner core. Cut into medium bite-sized pieces and place in a large bowl. To prepare cantaloupe and honeydew, slice the top and bottom off each fruit. Stand melons upright and cut off the outer skin. Cut in half and remove the inner seeds with a spoon. Cut into ¼ wedges and slice wedges into medium bite-size pieces. Place in bowl with pineapple. Remove tops from strawberries and slice into ¼ pieces. Remove outer skin from kiwi and cut into medium bite-size pieces. Combine pineapple, cantaloupe, melon, strawberries, and kiwi and toss all fruit together. Pour juice over fruit and serve in individual bowls.

Serving Size: 6

Tip: Some may ask, why add juice to fruit? The acidity in the juice allows the fruit to release its natural juices and provides additional sweetness to the salad.

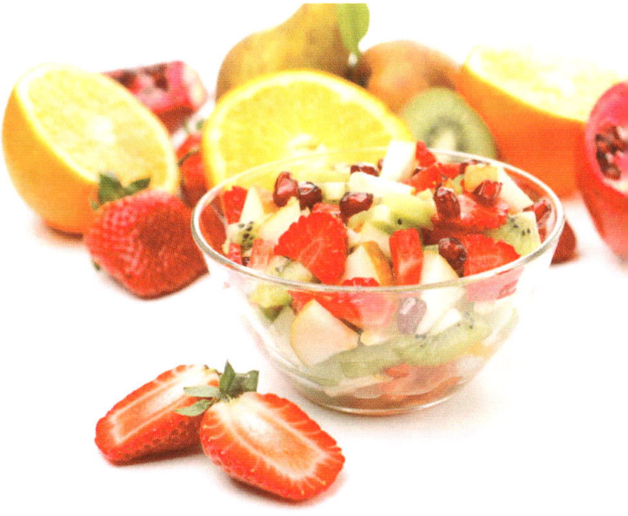

Peanut Butter Bars

¼ cup walnuts, finely chopped

½ cup raisins

¼ tsp. cinnamon

¼ cup old fashioned rolled oats

¼ cup sliced almonds, chopped

¼ cup dried cranberries

¼ tsp. nutmeg

½ cup smooth natural peanut butter

Instructions

Place prepared walnuts and almonds in a large bowl. Combine raisins, dried cranberries, and oats with walnuts and almonds. Add cinnamon and nutmeg and stir. Mix in the peanut butter, combining all ingredients together. Line an 8" x 8" x 2" glass pan with parchment paper and pour peanut butter mixture into pan, spreading evenly. Place pan in the freezer for 20-30 minutes or until the peanut butter bar mixture has hardened. Cut into bar-size pieces and remove parchment paper.

Tip: Specialty grocery stores have all-natural peanut or almond butter stands where you can grind your own nut butter. If you cannot find this in your store, be sure to use all-natural, no sugar added peanut butter for this recipe.

Serving Size: 8

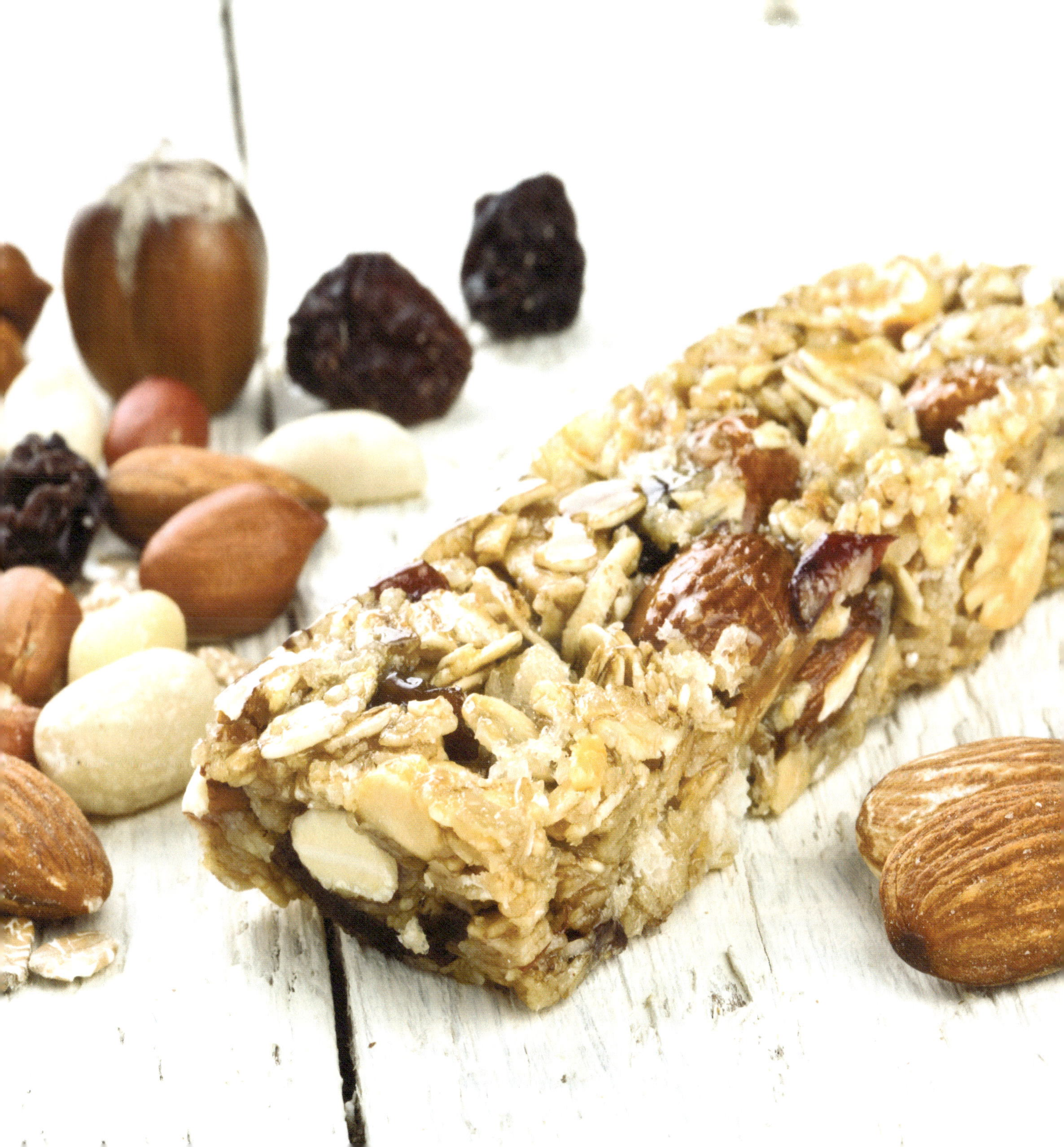

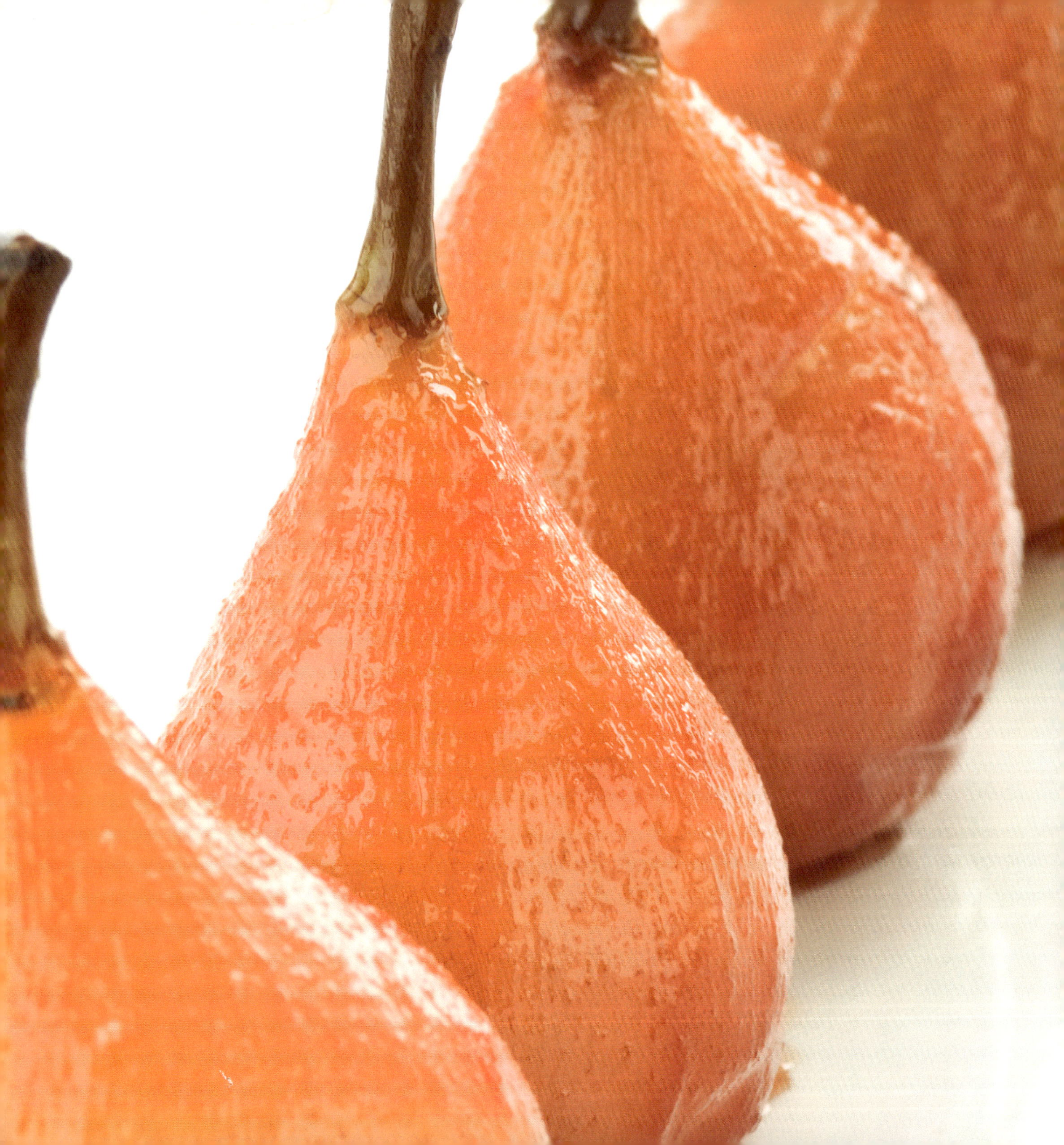

Poached Pears

2 Bosc pears, firm with stems attached

⅔ cup 100% pear juice

1 cinnamon stick

1 cup 100% orange juice

2 cups water

1 tsp. pumpkin spice

Instructions

Cut off bottom of pear; remove skin and set aside. In a large stockpot combine orange and pear juice, water, cinnamon stick, and pumpkin spice. Bring to a simmer and add pears, placed on their sides, in the poaching liquid. Allow pears to simmer for 25-30 minutes or until you can easily pierce them with the tip of a paring knife. Occasionally turn the pears over to allow for even cooking. When pears are done, transfer to a shallow serving platter. To make syrup from the poaching liquid, remove the cinnamon stick and raise the heat until the liquid boils. It will take approximately 15 minutes for the liquid to boil and reduce down. The result will be a thin syrup. You will need to stir the liquid occasionally to avoid burning. When poaching liquid is reduced to syrup, pour over top of pears.

Tip: It may be difficult to find 100% pear juice in the juice aisle of your grocery store. If you can't find it with the other juices, check the infant/toddler section.

Serving Size: 2

If you abide in Me, and My words abide in you, you will ask what you desire, and it shall be done for you. By this My Father is glorified, that you bear much fruit; so you will be My disciples. John 15:7-8

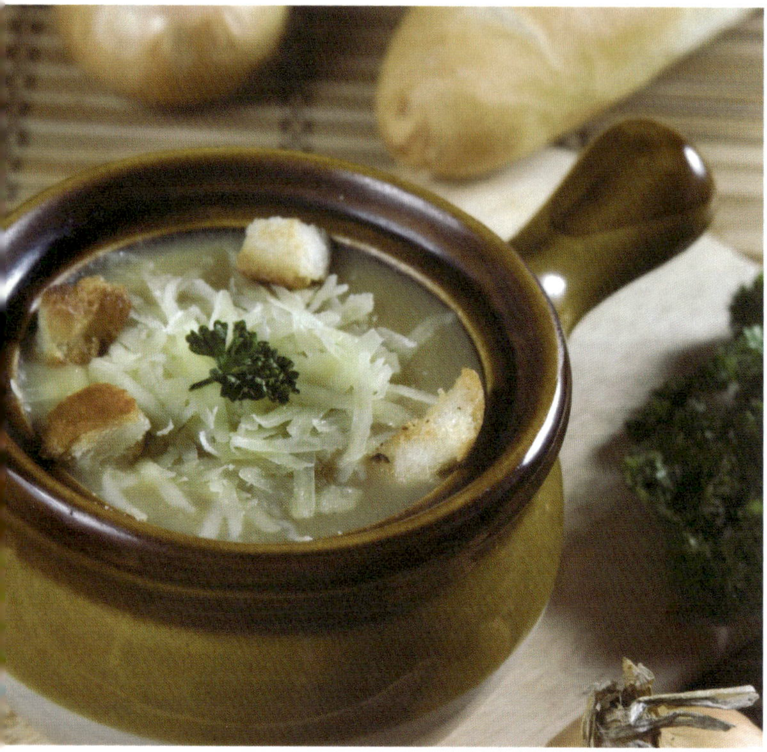

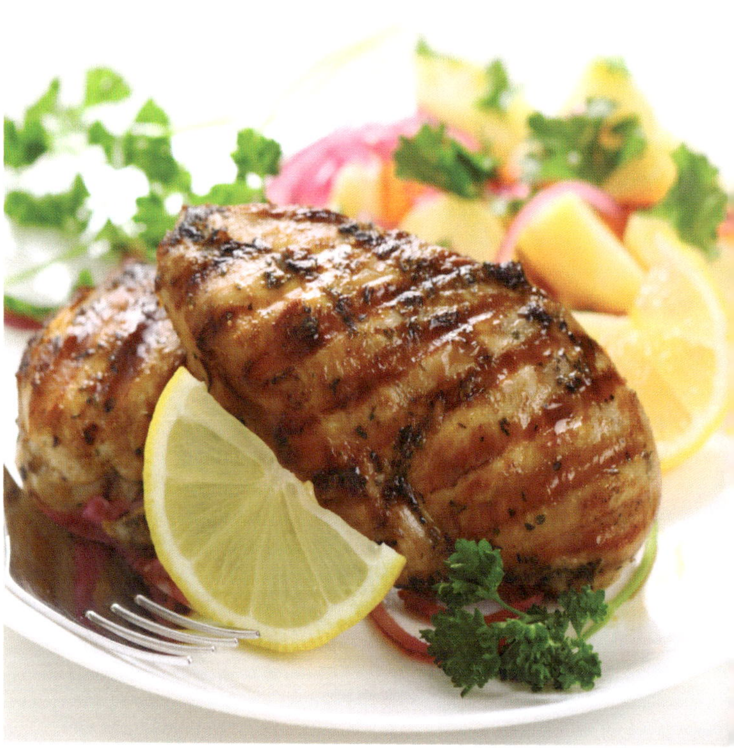

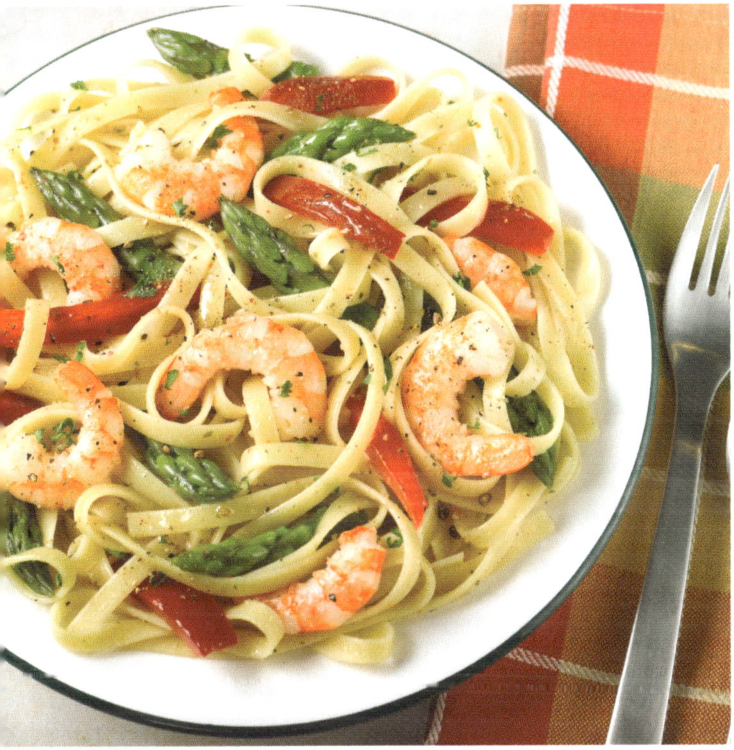

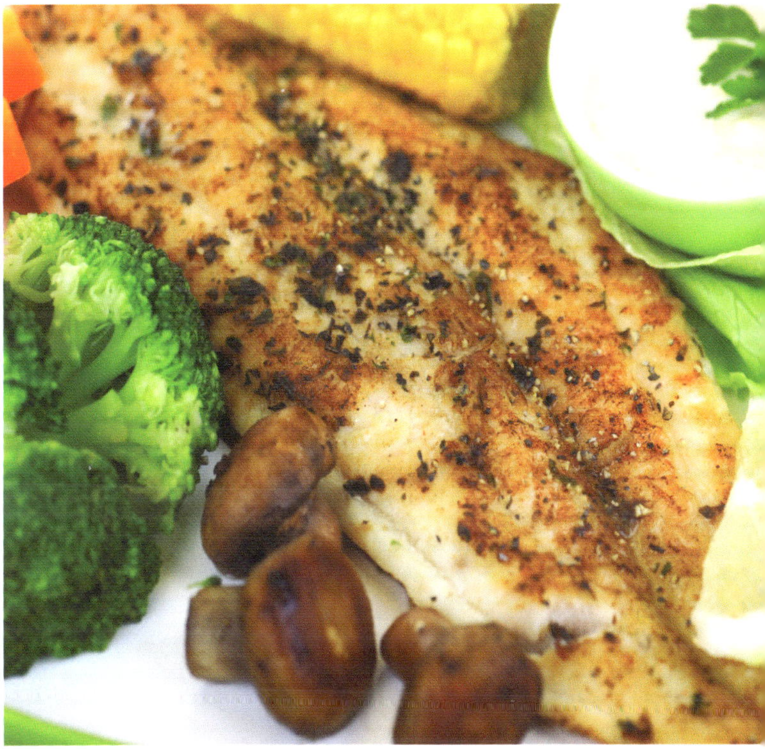

Post Daniel Fast

Tip: If you use a whole roasted chicken, remove the skin and de-bone the entire chicken. If you choose to use split chicken breasts, place them on an ungreased baking sheet. Season chicken with salt, pepper, and olive oil. Roast for 20 minutes at 350 degrees. Once chicken is cooked allow it to cool. Remove skin, de-bone and cut into bite-sized chunks.

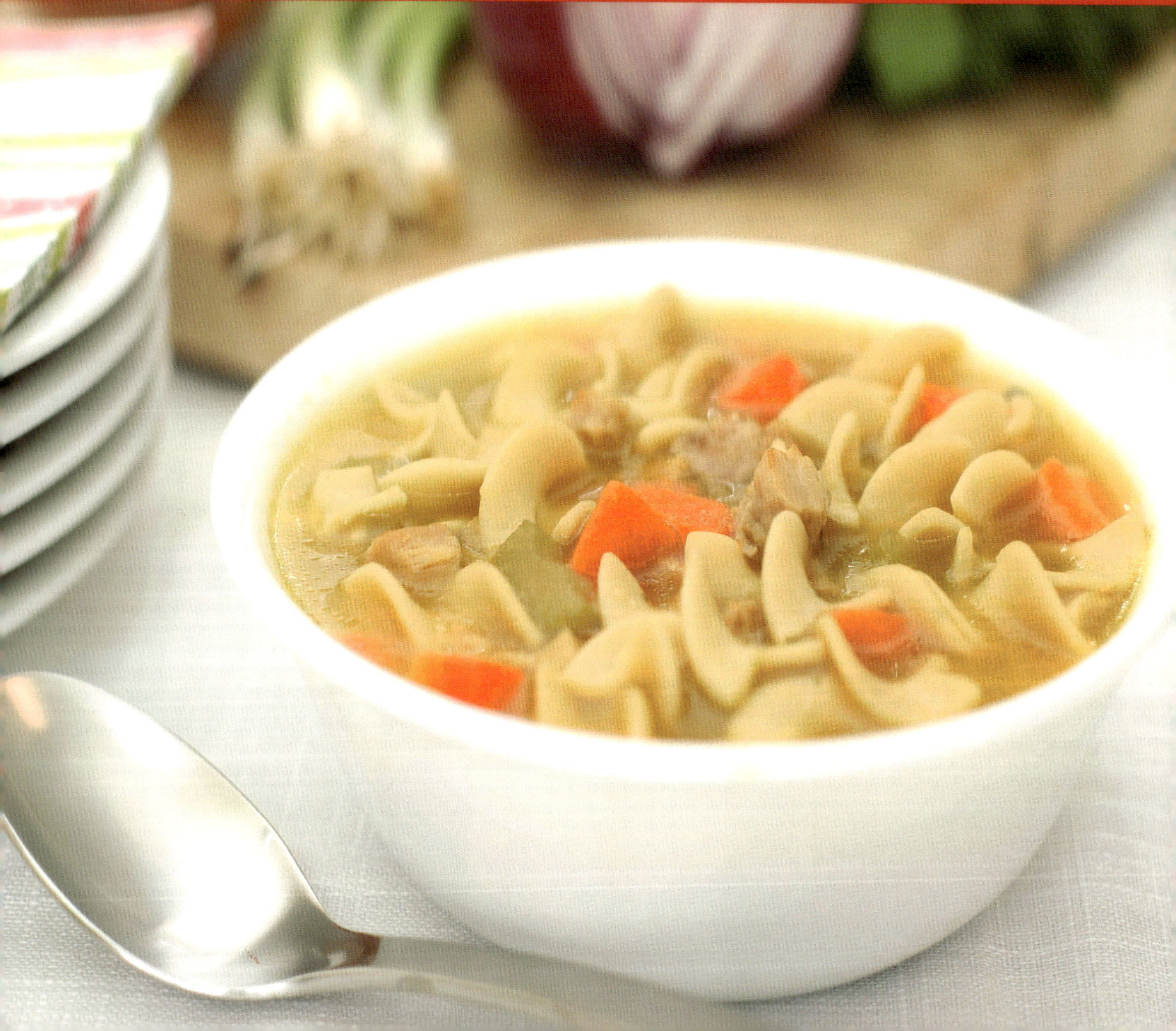

Chicken Noodle Soup

3 tbs. olive oil

½ tsp. black pepper

4 carrots, peeled and chopped

1 large onion, minced

3 chicken bouillon cubes

1 tbs. poultry seasoning

1 tsp. kosher salt

4 celery stalks, chopped

16 oz. chicken broth

8 cups water

3 chicken breasts or whole roasted chicken, cooked (see tip on page 136)

1 lbs. Kluski home-style noodles or egg noodles

Instructions

Chop onion, celery, and carrots into bite-sized pieces. Put olive oil, onion, celery, and carrots in a large stockpot. Cook over medium heat for approximately 10-15 minutes or until onions are translucent and celery and carrots are tender. Season with salt, pepper, and poultry seasoning. Add 4 cups of water and 2 chicken bouillon cubes to soup mixture and bring to a boil. Add half the bag of noodles to broth and cook according to package directions. When noodles are al dente, add the chicken to the mixture (see tip for chicken preparation instructions). Add the remaining 4 cups of water and 1 chicken bouillon cube. Simmer for 10 minutes.

Serving Size: 6

French Onion Soup

2 tbs. unsalted butter

¼ tsp. black pepper

2 cans beef consommé

1 French baguette, sliced

5 sweet Vidalia onions, thinly sliced

¼ tsp. kosher salt

1 box beef broth (32 oz.)

1 cup water

1 cup Gruyere cheese, shredded

Instructions

In a large sauté pan, melt butter over medium heat. Add onions, salt, and pepper. Sauté onions until caramelized; this will take approximately 15-20 minutes. Spoon caramelized onions into large stockpot and add water, beef broth, and beef consommé. Allow soup to simmer on medium-low heat for 30-45 minutes. Preheat oven to broil setting. Ladle prepared soup into an ovenproof soup bowl and place sliced French baguette rounds on top. Sprinkle 2 tablespoons of grated Gruyere cheese over each slice of bread. Place bowl on a baking sheet and set under broiler to melt and brown the cheese (approximately 1-2 minutes).

Tip: To quickly caramelize onions, add ½ tablespoons of sugar. The sugar will accelerate the caramelization process, resulting in sweeter onions.

Serving Size: 6

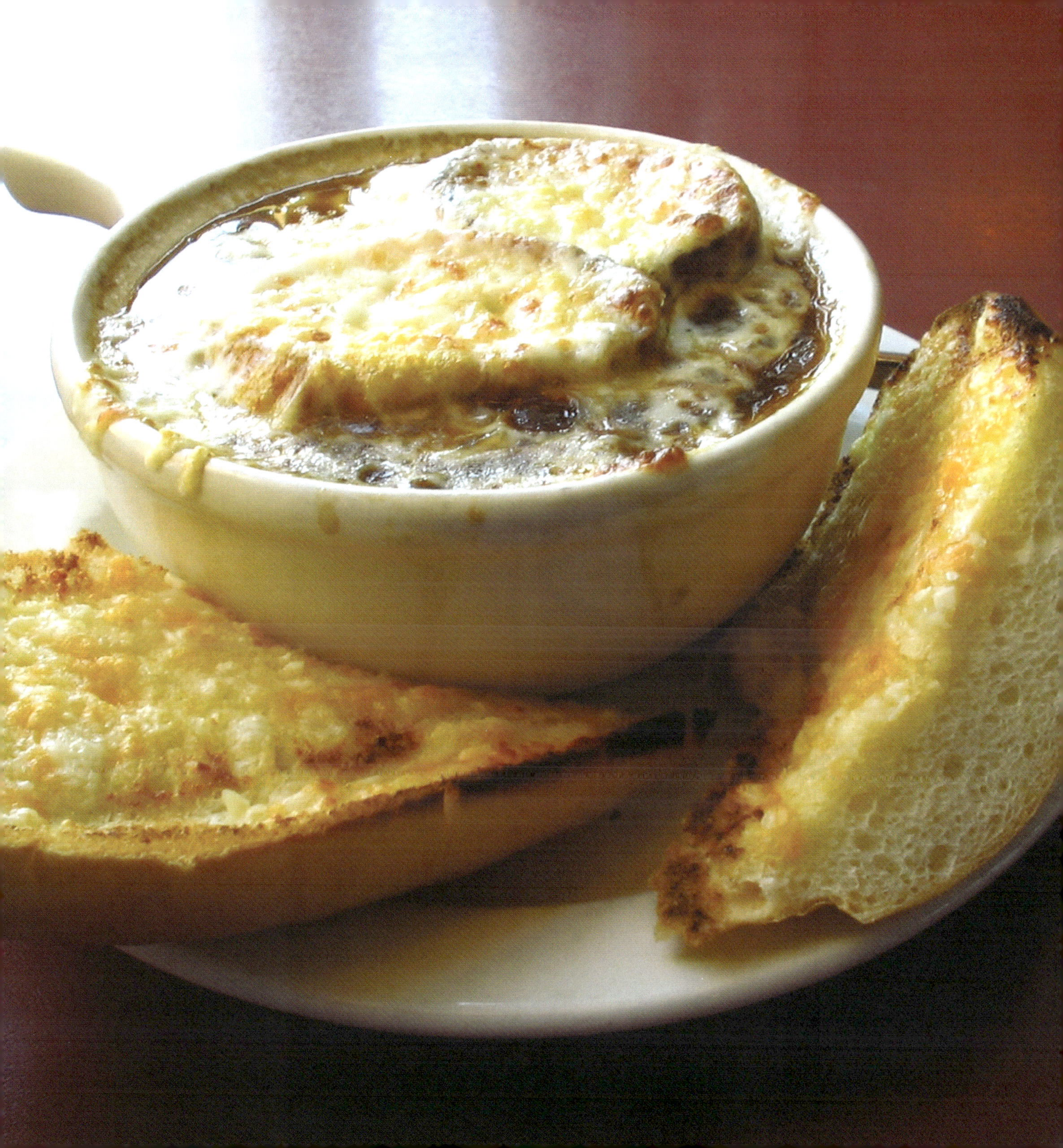

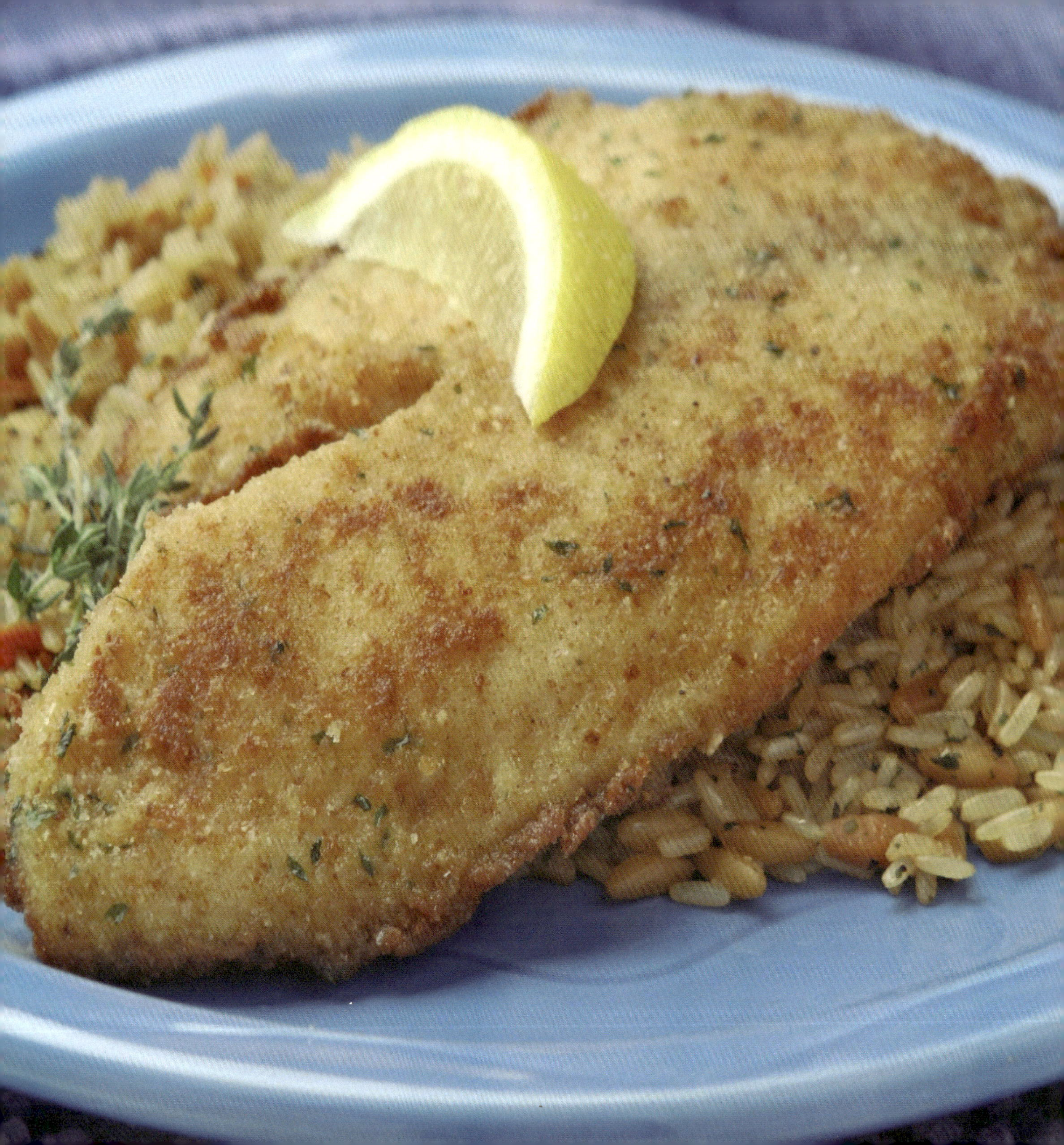

Pan Fried Cornmeal Tilapia

4 tilapia filets

1 tbs. Lawry's season salt

2 eggs

¾ cup peanut oil

1 cup yellow corn meal

1 tsp. black pepper

⅓ cup milk

Instructions

Season tilapia filets with season salt and pepper. In a separate bowl, beat the eggs and milk together. Dip tilapia in the egg and milk mixture, then into the yellow corn meal. Heat peanut oil in a medium sauté pan. Fry breaded tilapia filets to a golden brown, approximately 3-5 minutes on each side. Place fried fish on a paper towel to remove excess oil.

Tip: This breading recipe can be used on many different types of fish. I recommend trying the same process with perch or catfish.

Serving Size: 4

Shrimp & Broccoli Pasta with Garlic Butter Sauce

1 lb. spaghetti

3 garlic cloves, minced

1 ½ tsp. kosher salt

2 cups broccoli florets

1 stick butter, unsalted

1 shallot, minced

¼ tsp. black pepper

½ cup grated parmesan cheese

1 lb. medium frozen raw shrimp, shelled and de-veined (60-80 count)

Instructions

In a large bowl submerge frozen shrimp in cold water and thaw 5-7 minutes or until completely thawed. Drain water, remove tails and shell, and set aside. In a large stockpot boil spaghetti to al dente per package instructions. In a medium stockpot add ½ cup of water and broccoli florets. Bring water to a low simmer and add broccoli; steam for approximately 8-10 minutes. Place broccoli in a bowl of ice water to stop the cooking process, then strain and set broccoli aside. In a large skillet melt the butter over medium-high heat, add the chopped garlic and shallots, and cook 1-2 minutes or until shallots are translucent. Add shrimp to skillet with the melted butter and cook approximately 2-4 minutes per side, turning the shrimp over halfway through the cooking process. Add spaghetti and broccoli to the skillet and mix in the butter sauce. Add salt, pepper, and grated parmesan cheese to taste.

Serving Size: 4

Tip: For a quicker cooking process, use frozen microwaveable broccoli florets. Prepare broccoli as instructed on package and add to the pasta as instructed in the recipe.

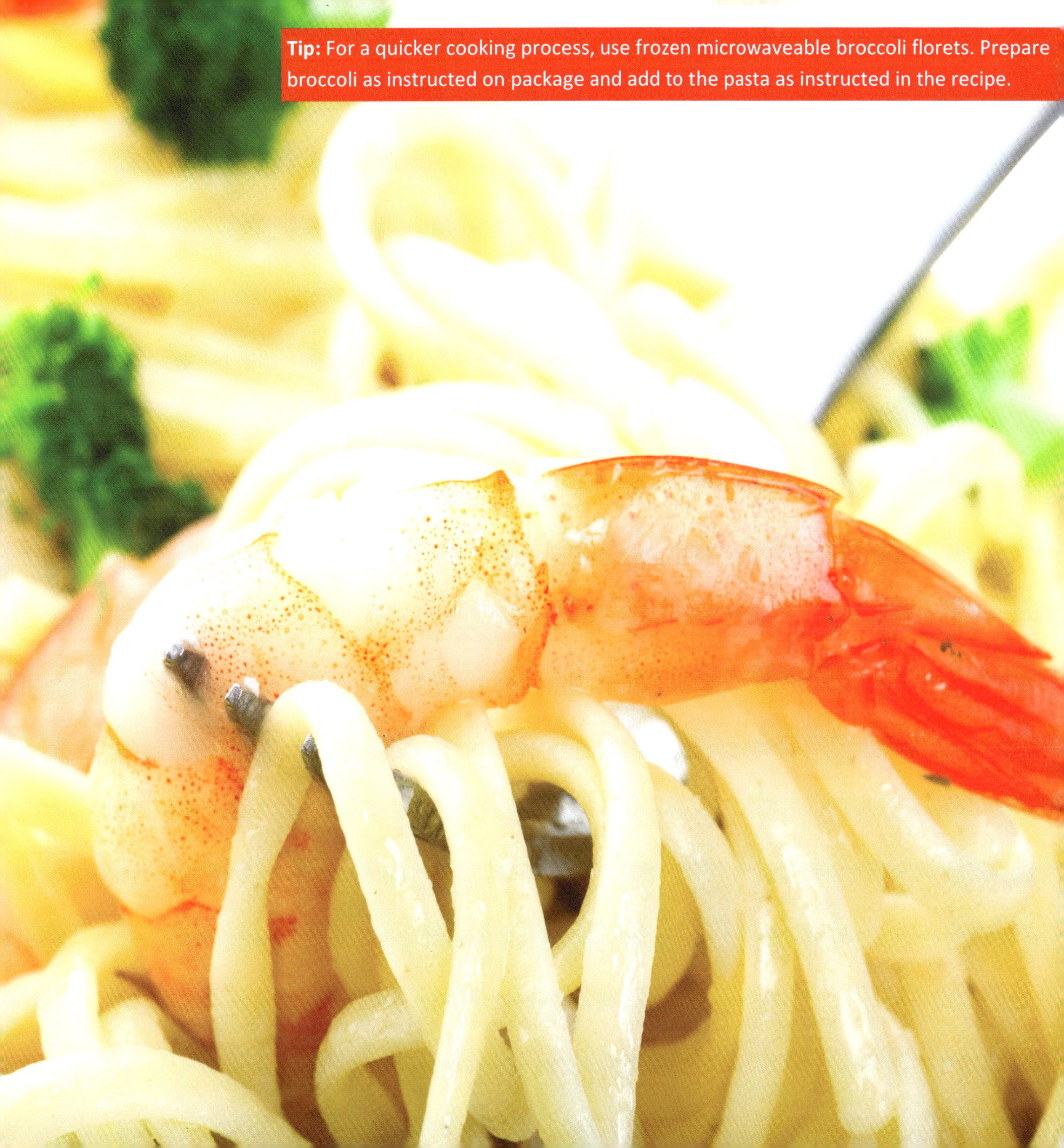

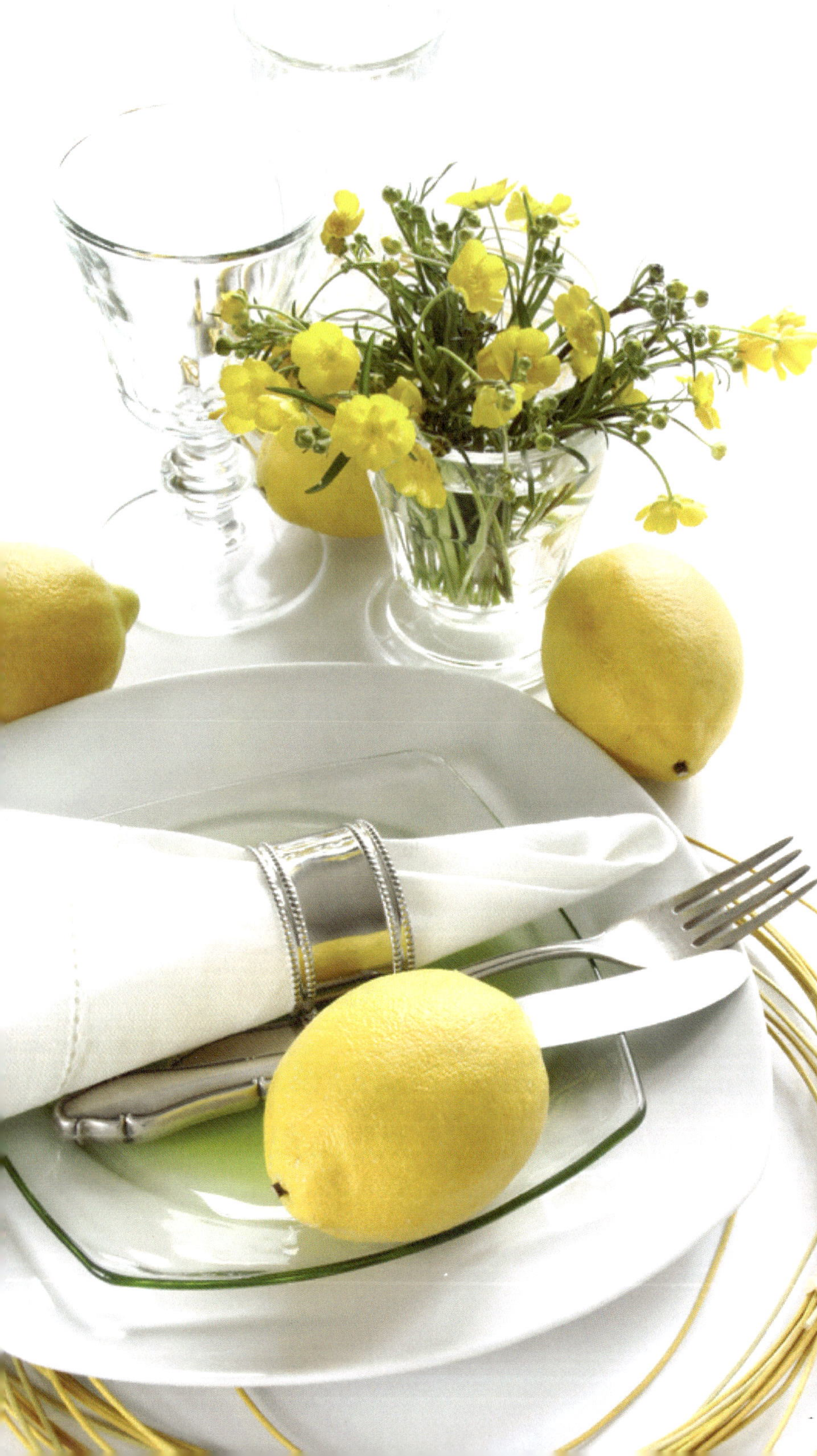

Fasting to Be Seen by God!

Matthew 6:16-18 NLT

And when you fast, don't make it obvious
as the hypocrites do, for they try to look
miserable and disheveled so people will
admire them for their fasting.
I tell you the truth, that is the only rewar
they will ever get. But when you fast,
comb your hair and wash your face.
Then no one will notice that you are
fasting, except your Father, who knows
what you do in private. And your Father,
who sees everything, will reward you.

Index

Index

Index

CPSIA information can be obtained
at www.ICGtesting.com
Printed in the USA
263197LV00002B